"This is an essential guide for patients living with arthritis and is indispensable for the family members, yoga professionals, and medical providers that care for them. As a physician, I find this book to be an excellent resource to better understand the whole-person approach to treating arthritis through yoga."

—*Dana DiRenzo, MD, MHS, Johns Hopkins Division of Rheumatology*

"*Yoga Therapy for Arthritis* is a groundbreaking resource for people living with arthritis and those who care for them. Combining research and education with yoga philosophy and practices, this book provides a user-friendly, comprehensive, empowering, whole-person approach to navigating the physical, mental, and spiritual challenges associated with arthritis. I highly recommend this book for individuals living with arthritis as well as medical, health, and yoga professionals."

—*Jennifer Kreatsoulas, PhD, E-RYT 500, C-IAYT, author of* Body Mindful Yoga

"*Yoga Therapy for Arthritis* offers valuable facts and compassionate insights honouring the whole being through deep understanding of the lived human experience beyond the muscles, bones and joints. Clear, engaging, and practical, this book is an informative and accessible toolbox for those who suffer, and for those who serve them, in the health and yoga profession."

—*Helene Couvrette, C-IAYT, E-RYT500, President of MISTY—*
Montreal International Symposium on Therapeutic Yoga

"*Yoga Therapy for Arthritis* offers yoga teachers, yoga therapists, healthcare practitioners, and the everyday person an innovative holistic perspective on the whole human experience of living with arthritis. The tone of the book is one of empowerment, hope, and compassion. It is a valuable resource that will inspire anyone living with arthritis, along with those that care for them personally and professionally. I highly recommend this book!"

—*Kristen Butera, E-RYT 500, C-IAYT, Program Director,*
Comprehensive Yoga Therapy, and author of Yoga Therapy:
A Personalized Approach for Your Active Lifestyle

"It is rare to find an author who can speak so expertly on the spiritual and on the physical—and that's exactly what Steffany Moonaz has done here. She is bridging a divide that is rarely crossed, and we all benefit from the intersection of truth, love, and wisdom found in this book."

Jivana Heyman, Founder of Accessible Yoga

YOGA
THERAPY
FOR ARTHRITIS

of related interest

Yoga Therapy for Stroke
A Handbook for Yoga Therapists and Health Care Professionals
Arlene A. Schmid and Marieke Van Puymbroeck
Forewords by Matthew J. Taylor and Linda Williams.
ISBN 978 1 84819 369 7
eISBN 978 0 85701 327 9

Yoga Therapy for Digestive Health
Charlotte Watts
ISBN 978 1 84819 354 3
eISBN 978 0 85701 312 5

Yoga Therapy for Fear
Treating Anxiety, Depression and Rage with the Vagus Nerve and Other Techniques
Beth Spindler
ISBN 978 1 84819 374 1
eISBN 978 0 85701 331 6

Yoga Therapy as a Creative Response to Pain
Matthew J. Taylor
Foreword by John Kepner
ISBN 978 1 84819 356 7
eISBN 978 0 85701 315 6

Principles and Themes in Yoga Therapy
An Introduction to Integrative Mind/Body Yoga Therapeutics
James Foulkes
Foreword by Mikhail Kogan, MD
Illustrated by Simon Barkworth
ISBN 978 1 84819 248 5
eISBN 978 0 85701 194 7

Yoga Therapy for Parkinson's Disease and Multiple Sclerosis
Jean Danford
ISBN 978 1 84819 299 7
eISBN 978 0 85701 249 4

Yoga for a Happy Back
A Teacher's Guide to Spinal Health through Yoga Therapy
Rachel Krentzman, PT, E-RYT
Foreword by Aadil Palkhivala
ISBN 978 1 84819 271 3
eISBN 978 0 85701 253 1

YOGA
THERAPY
FOR ARTHRITIS

A Whole-Person Approach
to Movement and Lifestyle

STEFFANY MOONAZ AND ERIN BYRON

Foreword by Dr. Clifton O. Bingham III, MD

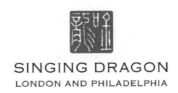

SINGING DRAGON
LONDON AND PHILADELPHIA

The poem on page 114 is printed with permission from Many Rivers Press, www.davidwhyte.com. David Whyte, Sweet Darkness © Many Rivers Press, Langley, WA USA.

First published in 2019
by Singing Dragon
an imprint of Jessica Kingsley Publishers
73 Collier Street
London N1 9BE, UK
and
400 Market Street, Suite 400
Philadelphia, PA 19106, USA

www.singingdragon.com

Library of Congress Cataloging in Publication Data
Names: Moonaz, Steffany, author. | Byron, Erin, 1973- author.
Title: Yoga therapy for arthritis : a whole-person approach to movement and
    lifestyle / Steffany Moonaz and Erin Byron.
Description: London ; Philadelphia : Jessica Kingsley Publishers, 2018. |
    Includes bibliographical references.
Identifiers: LCCN 2018019297 | ISBN 9781848193451
Subjects: | MESH: Arthritis--therapy | Yoga | Holistic Health | Life Style
Classification: LCC RC933 | NLM WE 344 | DDC 616.7/22062--
dc23 LC record available at https://lccn.loc.gov/2018019297

British Library Cataloguing in Publication Data
A CIP catalogue record for this book is available from the British Library

ISBN 978 1 84819 345 1
eISBN 978 0 85701 302 6

Printed and bound in Great Britain

In memory and appreciation of my dear mother, Cyndi Lee Haaz (1952–2018),
who lived by the most foundational principles
of yoga without even knowing it.

Steffany

Contents

Foreword by Dr. Clifton O. Bingham III, MD   *11*

Acknowledgements   *15*

Introduction   21

Activity List   *32*

Part I   **Living with Arthritis**   **35**

Chapter 1   What Is Yoga Therapy for Arthritis?   37

Chapter 2   Arthritis Is a Whole-Person Disease   59

Chapter 3   Yoga Is a Whole-Person Practice   74

Chapter 4   Yoga, the Physical Body, and Arthritis
                   (*Annamaya Kosha*)   89

Chapter 5   The Energy Layer (*Pranamaya Kosha*)   104

Part II   **Thriving with Arthritis**   **121**

Chapter 6   Arthritis and Energy Levels   123

Chapter 7   Pain in the Brain (*Manomaya Kosha*)   138

Chapter 8   Arthritis and a Healthy Mind   155

Chapter 9   Wisdom and Perspectives on Arthritis
             (*Vijanamaya Kosha*)   171

Chapter 10   Spirituality in Arthritis (*Anandamaya Kosha*)   186

Part III   Yoga Therapy Practices for Arthritis   **207**

Chapter 11   Yoga Therapy at Home   209

Chapter 12   Sequences for Specific Intentions   228

Chapter 13   Where to Go from Here   249

Appendix   *Adapting and Modifying Postures*   *271*

             Resources   *318*

             Endnotes   *321*

Foreword

"You need to be extra careful with your wrists when you are doing a down dog." This is not the usual advice a patient with arthritis would expect to hear from their rheumatologist, yet it reflects a more holistic approach that I have learned to use in helping people with arthritis maximize function and improve quality of life. I was once a sceptic myself. My medical training prepared me well to understand the pathobiology of disease and to apply evidence-based approaches to manage the underlying disease process of various forms of arthritis. But my training was sorely lacking in teaching a holistic approach to help patients negotiate how to live with a chronic condition like arthritis.

Fortunately, before I was too set in my ways, I had the good fortune to work with Steffany (Haaz) Moonaz as she started a project in our academic rheumatology practice to study the effects of a yoga program, specifically modified to address the concerns of people living with rheumatoid arthritis and osteoarthritis. I introduced the program to a number of my own patients, who enthusiastically agreed to participate. As the study proceeded, I had patients report back on the improvements that they were experiencing in areas such as self-confidence, appreciation and acceptance of limitations, improvements in strength and balance, and even reductions in pain and fatigue. After the study was over, many patients continued with home-based yoga practices, noting the importance of this in "grounding" their daily lives. One of my patients even went on to become a yoga instructor herself! As the study concluded and we analyzed the data there were definite improvements noted in multiple different aspects of health-related quality of life, physical fitness, and psychological health.

I worked with Steffany as she developed her doctoral thesis, serving as one of her clinical advisors and watched her develop appreciation for the special concerns of patients living with various forms of arthritis. She was inquisitive and always cautious. Since completing her dissertation, Steffany has gone on to develop the successful Yoga for Arthritis (YFA) Program, based on the work done at Hopkins. She has worked with NIH on additional studies, collaborated with research hospitals in New York City, and directs the research program at the Maryland University for Integrative Health (MUIH). I have given lectures for the last several years to the Yoga Therapy Master's program at MUIH, providing information on joint safety and collaborative care between patients, providers, and yoga professionals that is respectful of physical limitations and medical concerns. Steffany covers some of this content in her final chapter with helpful tips for patients, practitioners, and teachers on creating a collaborative relationship.

There are a number of misconceptions among medical professionals about yoga. Some may have the "image" of yoga as the svelte, uber-flexible, Lululemon-clad yogini engaged in some twisty bendy pose, usually with a beautiful beach or other vista in the background as seen on covers of yoga and lifestyle magazines. Others think about the physically demanding types of hot yoga, power yoga, and athletic yoga practices that are composed of rooms of twenty-somethings pushing the limits of athleticism, and sometimes causing injuries. Alternatively, or additionally, we may envision yoga being wrapped up in some new-age, chanting, meditative practice performed by people sitting tightly cross-legged on the floor. With only these images of yoga, it is hard to imagine that such a practice could possibly be safe or appropriate for people with arthritis.

In medicine one of our primary tenets is *primum non nocere*, or "First, do no harm." Likewise, in yoga a central tenet is related to *ahimsa* or non-harming. Throughout the book, this primary principle is emphasized again and again to the potential practitioner with arthritis, instructors, or other interested health care professionals. Awareness, respect, and acceptance of limitations is an important component of the overall approach and program.

In her book, Steffany is able to demystify yoga. She takes us back to its foundational underpinnings to reveal the ways in which yoga can become accessible to those living with arthritis. The Yoga for Arthritis program developed at Hopkins was broad in its scope, encompassing much more than asanas (poses) to integrate other arms of yoga that address aspects of emotional and spiritual health.

Her book is directed toward patients, yoga instructors, and health professionals, all of whom can benefit from the information within. Personal stories of people with arthritis who have engaged in a modified yoga practice are inspiring; many of these are truly stories of transformation. Some of these are my own patients who continue to practice yoga a decade later. Step-by-step instructions on modifications of specific yoga poses are easily understandable and help readers to better understand their underlying intention. Information on meditative and breathing practices emphasize the non-physical aspects of yoga that have great potential as parts of holistic care. Exercises through the book demonstrate basic yogic principles (e.g., breathing, concentration, meditation, relaxation) in addition to further information on stress reduction.

As I watched the changes in my patients who participated in the program, I began my own yoga practice. This has been an important part of my own self-care and tremendously beneficial through injuries and other life challenges. The lessons learned from watching Steffany and working with YFA have helped me to rehabilitate from a back injury on more than one occasion. In fact, one of my injuries occurred after I had laid off of a regular yoga practice for several months. The lessons of acceptance of current state and non-harming were important as I began a graded recovery. I was able to experience firsthand the value of the different aspects of yoga as part of my own healing, not only of my physical injury but also the associated social and emotional impacts of pain.

As a rheumatologist in practice for more than twenty-five years, I have seen thousands of patients with various forms of arthritis. One of the most inspirational aspects of caring for this unique patient population is witnessing the resilience embodied by many patients. Physicians now have tremendous therapies now available to help treat inflammation and autoimmune-driven aspects of a number of forms of arthritis. However, I have great appreciation for totality of bio-psycho-social impacts on health-related quality of life that extends far beyond the physical impacts of joint swelling and pain. Since my introduction to the yoga for arthritis program, I can now draw upon additional complementary tools to more holistically care for my patients. And as the health care system seemingly squeezes more and more time from our encounters, potentially compromising our ability to best treat the "whole patient," I see a sensible program incorporating the tenets of yoga as an important available adjunct for holistic care.

As health professionals increasingly understand the value of movement for people with arthritis, a properly modified yoga program can encourage movement, promote body awareness, improve flexibility, improve biomechanics, and strengthen periarticular structures (tendons, ligaments, muscles). Additionally, the mind-body aspects of yoga practice help to address psychosocial and spiritual aspects of disease, potentially helping to mediate pain pathways, improve self-efficacy, reduce stress, and encourage self-acceptance. The mechanisms through which yoga and meditation may exert their effects are still unclear and require further scientific study, but the value of physical activities and mind-body interventions is increasingly demonstrated through rigorous clinical studies.

The book that Steffany has written provides a wealth of information for a variety of audiences, written in a way that is accessible to all. This book will provide an introduction for individuals with arthritis seeking to learn more about participating in yoga, specific guidance for yoga professionals to use in modifying practices for individuals with arthritis, and demystification and helpful guidance for health professionals who are more interested in learning about the use of complementary approaches to better care for their patients. With the information from this book patients, yoga professionals, and health providers can collaboratively integrate a yoga practice as part of whole-person, patient-centered arthritis care, that includes evidence-informed complementary practices, promotes healthy lifestyle modifications, and improves self-care.

Clifton O. Bingham III, MD
Director, Johns Hopkins Arthritis Center
Deputy Director of Research, Division of Rheumatology
Professor of Medicine, Johns Hopkins University
Baltimore MD
August 2018

Acknowledgements

Steffany Moonaz, PhD, C-IAYT

In my pursuit to understand how mind and body interrelate to influence health and wellbeing, I work in an untraditional area of scientific inquiry. I thank all those who have been open-minded enough to consider the importance of bringing scientific rigor to mind-body modalities such as yoga, while remaining true to the origins of such practices. Looking closely at other views of healing can only enhance our clinical and methodological tools.

Thank you to all the participants in our yoga research, at Johns Hopkins Bayview, Good Samaritan Hospital, and the National Institutes of Health (NIH) for their willingness to face challenges and explore the range and the boundaries of their own movement and thinking. I have seen in you a tenacity and hope that is inspirational.

I thank the organizations that have funded and recognized our research over the past 15 years, including NIH/NCCAM (now NCCIH), the Arthritis Foundation, American College of Rheumatology, American Public Health Association, Johns Hopkins Bloomberg School of Public Health, International Association of Yoga Therapists, and the Maryland University of Integrative Health (MUIH).

Thank you James Snow, for seeking me out and bringing me to the tribe of MUIH when the Masters of Science in Yoga Therapy was only a plan and an institutional research agenda was only a dream. Thank you for believing in me and advocating for me, allowing me to take a leap of faith into my current academic home.

I thank the yoga therapy faculty and students at MUIH who were willing to welcome research into their course of study and were able to recognize the importance of our growing evidence-base. In particular, Diane Finlayson trained me as a yoga therapist, provided the space for my first teacher training, and now whole-heartedly champions my ongoing work. A deep bow of gratitude for it all. Marlysa Sullivan reminds me to stay excited about research and keep a fresh perspective about what is possible now and to come.

Thank you to Kimberly Middleton and Charlene Muhammad for taking this work to the next step, answering a question that was burning within me, and keeping Yoga for Arthritis squarely in the realm of public health. Our work matters most when it reaches those who struggle without access, without empowerment, without a voice at the table. I have been honored to work with you and to be a champion for diversity of all kinds in yoga and beyond.

Jennifer Daks and Christa Fairbrother nurtured Yoga for Arthritis from a one-woman show to an expanding organization with international reach. You have both been the glue that held our community together and helped me bring my work from the Ivory Tower to the lives of real people, forever changed by the practices of yoga. You serve as examples of what is possible in a life with arthritis. I am regularly inspired by you and thank you for sharing so much of yourselves in this work.

Thank you to all of the yoga teacher trainers and yoga teachers who do this work in their communities every day and provide a safe and welcoming place for people with arthritis to practice yoga. That was my dream and it has become a reality because of your caring and commitment to this work. Nancy O'Brien, Livvie Mann, and Peter Karow built and sustained a beautiful *sangha* of teachers in New York City, while Ann Swanson followed me to MUIH and has carried the torch of this work from there.

Thank you to everyone who was willing to share of themselves in the stories of this book. Some of you were in our research studies and showed me the humanity behind the data. Others of you are yoga teachers yourselves and teach this work from a place of deep personal understanding. Each of you helps this information to come alive in ways that I could never facilitate otherwise.

Erin Byron, this book would not exist without you. We shared a room at a yoga conference and when I mentioned my reluctance to write this book, you said, "I am only going to make this offer once…" and the rest is history. Thank you for making that offer, for holding my hand (because, boy, did I need it!), and for letting my work come through with my voice.

I thank Swami Satchidananda for leading me to the teachings of yoga and allowing me to explore what an Eastern guru can mean to a Western Jew. I also thank Rabbi Daniel Burg at Beth Am Synagogue for welcoming my comparisons between yogic and Jewish philosophy and for seeing them both as valid spiritual pursuits.

There are so many instances of serendipity or perhaps Divine intervention, and many people who knowingly or unknowingly connected dots along my path. At times, it has felt as though breadcrumbs fell before me and I was able to simply follow them on my journey. Thank you to the person who posted my résumé on a bulletin board in a hospital basement. Thank you to the person who first suggested I write about arthritis. Thank you to whoever and however the Big Magic happens for all of us who are willing to allow it. This includes the mentors in each stage of my journey. Melody Embry taught me to dance, which was my way into embodied mindfulness and sparked my early epiphany about its healing power. Nusha Martynuk encouraged me to explore the mind-body problem as both a scientist and an artist and has been a guiding light and a touchpoint ever since. Karen Bradley helped me to find and refine my eye and my voice as a writer and critic, which was a key to the discernment and critical thinking that science demands. Susan Bartlett welcomed an over-educated dancer into the Johns Hopkins Arthritis Center and taught me how to be a scientist both practically and culturally, without losing my passion and optimism. Larry Wissow was willing to work with me despite the difference in our research areas, allowing me to be the subject-matter expert, which is a role I have been fortunate to continue playing ever since. Clifton Bingham, (a.k.a. Bing), thank you for being willing to send your patients to me, for knowing that not all yoga is the same, and for sharing your perspective with my MUIH students who need to know that inter-professional communication *can* go both ways when we are all open-minded and willing to widen the tent in service to our common goal of serving others without harm.

Thank you to the team at Singing Dragon/Jessica Kingsley Publishers for finding me and giving me a chance to write my work for broader audiences than my research will ever reach otherwise. I love that yoga therapy has become a genre that publication houses would want to pursue. I appreciate the opportunity to write this from a whole-person perspective and not from the reductionism that many expect of the intersection between yoga and arthritis. Claire Wilson, Hannah Snetsinger, Daisy Watt, and Emily Badger—your support and efforts have been invaluable.

My family of origin is the buoy that keeps me afloat when the tide is high and the winds blow. No matter where those winds take me, I will always swim back to you. You have shown me how to be whole and live a life that is full, how to work and play with equal rigor, how to love and give with all of your heart and soul. What a legacy. Dad, thanks for giving me a job and letting me run away with it. Mom (1952–2018), you always insisted on living life to the fullest—having fun, working hard, loving, laughing, and being whole…cancer be damned, you showed me how to call the shots in my own life, whatever may come. MJ, my brother in all ways, cradle to grave and all along the way.

Soleil and Vie, the lights of my life. I am so honored to be a temporary guardian for your minds, bodies, and souls as you make your way in the world. I am inspired and humbled as I see you both becoming yourselves more firmly with each passing day. I hope that you grow up to see the world in beautiful ways that are beyond the scope of my imagination. If the effort I put into my work does nothing more than inspire you to reach for your dreams, it will be worth every moment. And perhaps I am able to bring some of what I have learned in this work to my connection with each of you. You were born yogis and I wish merely to help you to keep a spark of that alive within you, no matter what circumstances you may encounter.

To Rob—my darling, my soulmate, my partner in life and more, I could not have done this, any of this, without you. This leg of our journey has had its challenges, but it is made sweet by the sharing of it. We are eternal and eternally home together. Thank you for being my biggest fan, my greatest teacher, the other side of my coin, my fellow sojourner. I love you more, more, more.

Finally, I thank the Source of all life and all existence. May we all find the insight to see its spark within each other and all that surrounds us, for this is the beginning of a health and wholeness far beyond scientific measure. Namaste.

Erin Byron, MA, C-IAYT

Thank you to everyone who encouraged my learning and growth over all these years.

To my mom, Donna Byron, for tireless support in many forms. Your commitment to weightlifting and other forms of movement and exercise, inspires my own health. To her mom, my grandma Marie Elder and her sister Ruby Jackson for exhibiting acceptance and humor in the face of arthritic pain. To my father, Don Byron, for demonstrating the body's incredible power to heal itself and the importance of staying active and doing things you enjoy. To my brother, Kyle Byron, for continual inspiration towards healthy eating, movement, and self-care. To Susan

Charles for modeling strength and dedication. To Evelyn Lorraine Byron Charles for sweetening life.

To my partner Peter Arcari, I send thanks for your patience and understanding about the hours I spent on this book instead of helping you make salads. To Joshua Arcari for the professional support and uplifting presence. To Nathan Arcari for telling it like it is with gentleness, humor, and simplicity.

To Steffany Moonaz, my valued coauthor and the brilliant mind behind Yoga for Arthritis: thank you for your contributions to the field of yoga for arthritis research, yoga therapy, and integrative health. Thank you for taking a chance on me and trusting me with this big part of your life's work. I appreciate your diligence, creative gifts, and powerful sense of humor.

To my mentor, colleague, and friend Robert (Bob) Butera—thank you for leading by example and teaching me the essence of a yoga life. To the Yoga Institute of Mumbai for authentic teachings in tradition, self-reliance, and the ease of a pure practice. To my buddy Kristen Butera for inspiration as a mover and an author. To my Comprehensive Yoga Therapy Training co-faculty and honorary Canadian Staffan Elgelid, thanks for the perspectives and for always being at the ready with a joke.

To Marlysa Sullivan, thank you for recommendations and consultations. We used all those shoulder cues! Helene Couvrette, thank you for the Montreal International Symposium on Therapeutic Yoga and setting the stage for Steffany and I to collaborate! To my friends and colleagues of the International Association of Yoga Therapists, thank you for the work you do to bring integrity to the field of yoga therapy. To all of my yoga buddies.

To the many teachers who dedicated their lives to realized wisdom through daily practice, thank you for sharing your true discoveries. To my yoga therapy colleagues, thank you for your dedication to moving the field forward with integrity, clarity, and respect for tradition. To the many students I've encountered over the years and the many I'm about to meet, thank you for teaching me every single day. This thankfulness is most notable to the Friday noon Therapeutic Yoga students at Welkin YogaLife Institute, who were diligent in attending and keeping the yoga going in everyday life for many years, and taught me a great deal about arthritis in its many forms.

To the team at Singing Dragon/Jessica Kingsley Publishing. Claire Wilson, Hannah Snetsinger, Daisy Watt, and Emily Badger, you made this experience a genuine pleasure.

To the Brantford Community Symphony Orchestra, our long-suffering conductor Deb McLoughlin (who always meets us with a joke, no matter how many 3a.m. rehearsals), our dear departed founder Karl Langton, and each musician who keeps me smiling and inspired. To Emily and Michael Piekny for modeling possibility during an important time.

To everyone else who has influenced, supported, and encouraged me—I thank you. You know who you are and I appreciate you!

Disclaimer

The exercises in this book are in no way to be considered as a substitute for consultation with a medical practitioner, and should be used solely at the reader's discretion in conjunction with approved medical treatment. The author and the publisher are not responsible for any harm or damage to a person, no matter how caused, as a result of following any of the suggestions in this book.

INTRODUCTION

Yoga Therapy for Arthritis is a book for people living with arthritis and those who care for them. In addition to people affected by arthritis directly, healthcare professionals and yoga professionals will benefit from the research, practices, and personal stories included in this book.

Arthritis is not one single disease, but a category of over 100 different medical conditions. All of these different forms of arthritis are connected by the involvement of joint tissue. This often includes pain, stiffness, inflammation, and damage to joint cartilage and surrounding structures. Consequently, joints may be weakened, become unstable, or even deformed. Some types of arthritis, such as rheumatoid arthritis (RA), are systemic, meaning that the whole body is affected. For individuals with systemic forms of arthritis, other organs and body systems may be compromised, such as heart, lungs, kidneys, blood vessels, and skin. Arthritis can be so debilitating that in the United States, it is the leading cause of disability. It affects the whole person through pain, fatigue, increased health expenses, and changes in ability, employment status, and relationships (with themselves and others). People are simultaneously required to depend on others more and spend less time with them socially due to fatigue and other symptoms. Increased discomfort, limitation, self-perception, and isolation are very stressful. The external impairments are often more distressing than the pain, which can be intense. Sadly, many people with arthritis believe there is nothing that can be done to help them improve physically, energetically, emotionally, mentally, socially, and spiritually. That definitely is not the case!

Yoga is a no-impact mind-body activity with the potential to affect each of these levels of a person in some way. Yoga accommodates individual differences in ability and mobility and can be a safe and feasible form of physical activity for persons with arthritis. Yoga therapy offers improvements throughout the biopsychosocial-spiritual (BPSS) realms. The existing research on yoga for arthritis shows that it is safe and feasible for people with arthritis. A variety of demographics gain benefit from a range of yoga styles and intervention durations. Yoga has broad appeal and can be implemented in a variety of ways to increase physical fitness and mental health, in addition to reducing arthritis-related symptoms such as pain, tenderness, swelling, stiffness, and perhaps even systemic inflammation. Yoga postures help amplify strength, balance, flexibility, and endurance while strengthening tissues around the joints to further stabilize them. Practices such as mindfulness, breathing exercises, relaxation, and meditation, in addition to yoga philosophy and ethics, contribute to body awareness, improved mood, and decreased depression and anxiety, all while promoting stress resilience, acceptance of limitations, greater self-care, and enhancing self-efficacy for disease management. There is more engagement in life, activities, relationships, and service. The soul itself does not have arthritis; the disease may actually impel a journey that supports people in connecting to the deepest aspects of themselves and value the most important things in life.

Yoga therapy can also affect perceptions of overall wellbeing. It is particularly important for people with chronic conditions to learn positive ways of living with disease. Since people's perceptions of the severity of their arthritis is only weakly linked to overall health, there is increasing interest in assessing disease impact from the individual's viewpoint. As a mind-body activity, yoga therapy addresses aspects of physical and mental health. It has been shown to improve a range of quality of life and health measures. Furthermore, attending yoga classes improves people's social and spiritual wellbeing, while inspiring more strident self-care.

The approach described in *Yoga Therapy for Arthritis* includes structural adaptations, breathing practices, mental techniques, and other practices. This book also goes beyond those in-class approaches, to address how yoga therapy can reduce pain and have a positive impact on the whole person's BPSS wellbeing and overall quality of life. Through shifts in perspective and lifestyle, yoga therapy assists people with arthritis in cultivating deeper meaning, joy, and purpose. *Yoga Therapy for Arthritis* supports people in living differently with their disease.

Who Is This Book For?

This book teaches medical, health, and yoga professionals to support clients with rheumatic conditions, while guiding people living with arthritis to use their whole healthcare team as they pursue better self-care. We hope the book is inspiring to people with arthritis and teaches professionals how to appropriately apply yoga practices and philosophy. *Yoga Therapy for Arthritis* is written for anyone who is interested in arthritis and yoga—for any reason! Read on to understand more about the whole-person experience of living with arthritis and how the tools of yoga might be applied to improve physical, mental, social, and spiritual wellbeing.

Individuals living with the many conditions considered to be part of rheumatology (rheumatoid arthritis (RA), osteoarthritis (OA), lupus, gout, psoriatic arthritis, juvenile idiopathic arthritis, ankylosing spondylitis, and more) and those who love them, will benefit from reading *Yoga for Arthritis*. Individuals with arthritis might be most interested in the short practices that are scattered throughout the book or in the recommendations for how to find an appropriate yoga therapist/teacher and how to establish a home practice.

Arthritis is the leading cause of disability in the United States, and a better understanding of the challenges in life with arthritis can help foster compassion and support from individuals and communities touched by these conditions. Friends and family members might want to learn more about what it means to have arthritis, the many ways it can impact daily life, as well as the stories of transformation that show how real people have been able to live differently with their arthritis, no matter their age or diagnosis.

This book is a useful guide for yoga professionals, including yoga teachers and therapists. We hope that you are able to make use of the entire book from cover to cover. Arthritis is a primary reason students seek yoga as part of healthcare. Whether or not you specialize in working with musculoskeletal issues, autoimmune conditions, mental health, fatigue, accessibility, gentle yoga, chair yoga, or yoga for the general public, chances are you are already seeing students/clients with arthritis. The practice of yoga is becoming increasingly prevalent; the science regarding the benefits of yoga is becoming more robust and more people are turning to yoga as a part of their self-care and healthcare. Even if arthritis is not their reason for seeking yoga, arthritis is so prevalent that as yoga becomes more inclusive and available, you will be seeing more people living with the disease. The better you can understand it holistically, the better you can meet your students and clients where they are—with compassion, presence, and whole-person care. We intend for this book to help you understand arthritis in its many forms and how your tools can be best applied to help reduce suffering for those who seek your guidance.

Yoga Therapy for Arthritis is also written for medical professionals who work with arthritis patients of any kind. You are familiar with arthritis and rheumatic diseases and may therefore be most interested in the scientific bases for yoga as a component of arthritis management. Healthcare workers may find the research evidence useful in guiding recommendations and discussions with arthritis patients. While the biology of arthritis is very familiar to you, and you are likely also aware of how arthritis impacts all areas of life, short medical visits do not always provide the opportunity to hear about the transformational thinking that can happen in the context of these conditions. I invite you to read this with openness to possibility. Your tools are absolutely essential for improving the lives of patients with arthritis and related conditions. The tools of yoga may offer something complementary. You may have concerns about whether yoga can be safe and appropriate for all your patients, or some patients in particular. Those are valid concerns and are crucial for guiding patients toward appropriate resources and teaching. Not all yoga is the same and not all yoga is right for all patients. We hope that by the end of this book, you will feel more comfortable discussing yoga with your patients in an informed and supportive manner that aligns our shared intentions of non-harming and patient-centered care.

Authors' Stories

Steffany Moonaz, PhD, C-IAYT

I've been a dancer all of my life. My mother was a dance teacher during my childhood and I started classes at age three. I spent most evenings at the dance studio in classes and rehearsals of all kinds and spent my summers at performing arts camps—over the objections of my father's wallet! He urged me to try something different but none of the other arts had the same effect for me as dance did.

I noticed at a young age that something transformed for me in the dance studio. Whatever challenges I was having would melt away as soon as I started to dance. I would now call that "embodied mindfulness" or "mindful movement." When I danced, I was completely present in my body, without concern for past or future events. I remember thinking that this experience was a widely unknown gem. I knew that if more people experienced this feeling, there would be less suffering in the world.

I figured that whatever was happening for me in the studio must be happening in my brain and I intended to understand it better so that I could harness it to help people in suffering. I decided to major in neuroscience. But I soon discovered that neuroscience in the 1990s was less about directly helping people and more about mouse experiments. As a vegan, that quickly drove me to the biology department instead. But again, the dance department called to me. I graduated from Oberlin College with majors in biology, dance, and the pre-medical coursework to become a doctor. My honors thesis was about the physical, mental, and spiritual effects of dance. This was the beginning of my formal exploration into the mind-body connection, through the arts *and* the sciences.

I decided that I wanted to work with people directly, in some kind of healing capacity, but I also realized that I had some maturing to do. So, after a year of clinical research, I headed back to school for a Master of Fine Arts in dance. This, of course, was of great concern to my parents but I assured them that I still intended to become a doctor…eventually.

During my graduate studies, I explored the trappings of our increasingly sedentary lifestyle and the loss of expressive movement as a part of daily life. I organized spontaneous performances in public spaces, taught schoolchildren to dance around their desks, and even forced my own immediate family to join me on stage. Again, I was exploring ways to shift culture and encourage people to find the joy in mindful movement.

While in graduate school, I wanted to keep up the science on my résumé and looked for summer opportunities. During my first summer, I asked my father to share my résumé with anyone he knew who might have an opening. My résumé ended up posted on the corkboard in the basement of a building at Johns Hopkins University and my CMA (certified movement analyst) sparked the interest of a gastroenterologist. I was hired mainly to assist with bench research looking at esophageal cancer cells in culture with herbs, but she also asked me to apply my movement analysis skills to a sacred Bulgarian dance called Paneurythmy.

At my desk one day, the gastroenterologist suggested that I write a literature review about the effects of movement on RA. This is odd because she was a gastroenterologist, not a rheumatologist, and also because I knew *nothing* about RA at the time. But, I gave it a shot. There were six published studies at the time—two of dance, two of tai chi, and two of yoga. I wrote the paper and forgot about it. That doctor also told me that Moses is my spirit guide, and that my mission, like his, is to free people, but in a different way. (More on that later…)

The summer after graduating, I became a yoga teacher. Mind you, this was really only supposed to be for my own personal benefit. I had been practicing yoga and wanted to deepen my practice through a teacher training. I ended up at an ashram for a summer and right before I left, I came across my RA review paper. On a whim, I sent it to the Johns Hopkins Rheumatology Department with an explanation that I really knew nothing about RA and wanted to know if I should delete the paper or try to do something with it.

I got a phone call from a junior faculty member in rheumatology, a research psychologist named Susan Bartlett, who invited me in for a meeting. She was married to an exercise physiologist but had always hated exercise. Recently, she had tried her first yoga class and didn't distract herself just to get it over with. She actually wanted to be present and enjoy the experience. She felt that this could benefit arthritis patients and asked where I was in my studies.

By that point, I had discovered public health and realized it was a better path than medical school to help change the culture around mindful movement. I told her that I hoped to pursue a PhD in public health, but that I needed a break from school. As it turned out, her research assistant was leaving and she offered me a position where we would work on a study exploring the effects of yoga for RA. I could start taking classes at the Johns Hopkins Bloomberg School of Public Health, which she assured me was "the best public health school in the country." So, of course, that's exactly what I did. I went to live at an ashram for the summer and returned to join the Johns Hopkins Department of Rheumatology.

During my time at the ashram, I studied in the tradition of Dr. Dean Ornish, who discovered that yoga practices can reverse heart disease. At the ashram, Dr. Sandra (Amrit) McClanahan suggested that I could become "the Dean Ornish of arthritis," which is a humbling aspiration. I also had a profound experience in meditation while at the ashram. I discovered that I really wanted my life's work to help people experience more joy. It could be the mission the gastroenterologist foretold. Perhaps, then, my purpose is to help free people from whatever interferes with living more joyfully. Since arthritis is the nation's leading cause of disability, that seemed like a reasonable place to start. I returned to the Bloomberg School of

Public Health with a lofty goal aligned with the school motto of "Changing Lives, Millions at a Time," or maybe just a dozen at a time.

Dr. Bartlett had already received a bit of funding for a yoga pilot study when I arrived. I started teaching classes at the hospital right away and was learning a lot about how to adapt the practice to the RA population. I was also working on several other studies in the department. I led weight loss groups for people with knee OA and helped with studies of medication adherence, strength building, and social support. I attended Rheumatology Rounds at the hospital and learned about lupus, scleroderma, and ankylosing spondylitis. By working as a research assistant, I started to understand what would become my target population for many years to come.

The early 2000s was a good time for yoga research. The NIH National Center of Complementary and Alternative Medicine (NCCAM) had its biggest budget to date and yoga was getting a lot of interest. I received research funding from NCCAM, the Arthritis Foundation, the American College of Rheumatology, Johns Hopkins, and more. In fact, we received every grant we applied for during my seven years in the department, which Dr. Bartlett kept reminding me was very unusual… and would eventually stop. But during those years, we were able to expand the yoga study to both RA *and* OA, add a second location and a second yoga teacher, and expand the outcome measures. The study, which became the subject of my doctoral dissertation in public health, had grown in size, in rigor, and in duration. In fact, even many years later, it stood as the largest and most rigorous study of yoga in arthritis patients.

During the years that we conducted that study, I presented our work at many scientific conferences and received a lot of requests for interviews from journalists. As articles were published about our work in progress, my name became associated with the topic of yoga for arthritis. Thus, I started getting calls and emails from two groups: the first were people living with arthritis who wanted to know where to find an appropriate yoga class or instructor and the second were yoga teachers who wanted to know how to work safely with the arthritis patients coming into their classes. I felt a responsibility to address both sets of concerns.

The summer after I graduated with a PhD in public health, I spent a long weekend training six yoga teachers to work more safely with this population. That was the first of many such trainings in a dozen cities around the US, resulting in a growing workforce of yoga professionals who are equipped to meet the unique needs and limitations of students with various forms of arthritis.

YOGA THERAPY FOR ARTHRITIS

On the research side, I was contacted by an investigator from NIH Nursing who was interested in the feasibility of yoga for underserved minority populations with arthritis, both African American and Spanish-speaking. For the past several years, we have been exploring the replication of our initial research protocol for those populations, as well as some individuals with lupus.

In 2012, as the International Association of Yoga Therapists formalized the release of educational competencies for yoga therapists, the Provost from the Maryland University of Integrative Health saw an opportunity to develop a Masters of Science in Yoga Therapy. Based on my research and yoga teacher trainings for arthritis, I was one of the initial three faculty members for that program and have been teaching and conducting research at the university ever since.

In recent years, awareness has also broadened regarding the 300,000 children living with arthritis in the US. While there is not yet data to support the role of yoga for the management of juvenile idiopathic arthritis (JIA), both children with JIA and their parents are looking for tools that might help. I have been working with JIA patients from the ages of 2 to 22 and hope that research funding becomes available to explore age-appropriate yoga practice for that population.

I have been asked to write a book on yoga therapy for arthritis for many years, as one of the few people conducting research and education in this area. I have resisted that urging for a long time because there are already so many books about how to modify yoga poses. I just didn't think that another such book was needed, nor did I think it would be interesting to create. However, the more I talk about this work with yoga professionals, medical professionals, and people living with arthritis, the more I realize that there is a different book to be written. Arthritis is not a condition that only affects the joints. It affects the whole person. Similarly, yoga is not a practice that addresses only the joints. It addresses the whole person. The book that has not been written is the book about a whole-person approach to arthritis, through the whole-person practices of yoga.

In my 13 years of working in this area, I have seen much suffering. I hope this book furthers my mission of bringing greater freedom to the lives of people with arthritis because I have also seen much joy, discovery, and transformation. Sometimes those transformations are physical. Sometimes they start with something physical but end up impacting mental and emotional health. Sometimes the transformation is a complete shift in perspective about body, disease, or even life itself. The data is already published. I will share some of those findings in this book: how markers of physical and mental health improve with yoga practice and the science that can explain those changes. The stories behind that data have not been shared. It is my hope that through this book, readers will come to understand more about the human side of life with arthritis, and how life with arthritis can change—whether or not the arthritis actually changes. The data is powerful but the stories are even more so…and I promise to throw in some pose modifications, too, just for good measure.

The tagline at my *alma mater* of Johns Hopkins Bloomberg School of Public Health is "Saving Lives, Millions at a Time." There are millions of people living with arthritis. Whoever you are, you know some of them. This book will not *save* lives, but our hope is that it might *change* lives for the better by helping people with arthritis and those close to them see the distinction between pain and suffering, and addressing them both with the best that science and humanity can offer.

Erin Byron, MA, C-IAYT

I first met Steffany Moonaz when I attended her lecture on Yoga for Arthritis at the Montreal International Symposium on Therapeutic Yoga. At the time, I had been teaching yoga and providing yoga therapy sessions for nearly 20 years. That day, I was on an information-gathering mission for my mom, who has lived with OA for many years. Her mom also had arthritis and though she rarely complained, we all knew that Grandma's spine gave her constant trouble.

While listening to Steffany's presentation, I could relate much of what she said to my own approach with yoga therapy clients. Her compassionate perspective and strong scientific basis are highly engaging and inspiring. When she spoke of RA, I remembered Grandma's sister, Aunt Ruby, whose hands were so gnarled they were nearly useless to her for the last 20 years of life. I thought of myself and how yoga may support me in living with whatever genetic fate I may face as I continue to age. Steffany's research showed many opportunities to avoid greater damage from arthritis and ways that people living with rheumatic conditions can work with their experience of pain, depression, isolation, and functional limits.

I was honored when Steffany offered me the opportunity to delve more deeply into this topic and be a part of this book. Most of my contributions involve the philosophical and mental health components. Because *Yoga Therapy for Arthritis* is Steffany's life work and the content arises from her genius, it is written in her voice.

How to Use This Book

This book approaches arthritis (in its many forms) as a whole-person condition and presents yoga as a whole-person approach to disease management. It starts with a physiological perspective of why yoga may help in the management of arthritis. Arthritis is often falsely considered to be a disease of the musculoskeletal system only, and yoga is often considered to be merely a form of physical exercise for strengthening and stretching the physical body. This section will be of particular interest for those who are considering yoga as one of many available options for staying active with arthritis, which is important across conditions and through various stages of disease. But one should not stop there. The next section moves into the impact of arthritis on the levels of mind and emotion, which are impacted by arthritis and can be managed with yoga practices as a part of integrative care. Arthritis is a life-long, unpredictable, and challenging disease. Addressing the mental/emotional aspects of arthritis can impact the overall experience of the condition. *Yoga Therapy for Arthritis* considers higher aspects of meaning and purpose as they pertain to life with arthritis. Part II also expands the role for yoga practice in those regards. It is in this spiritual realm where we tend to see the most profound transformations and where we hope readers might be moved and inspired. Lastly, the book provides a series of concrete ways to apply the information. There are a range of sequences readers can practice at home and guidance on how to select an appropriate yoga class, teacher, and therapist.

Throughout this book, I offer practices and personal reflections to help manage rheumatic conditions. Please obtain clearance from your physicians and other healthcare providers before embarking upon this program. I recommend that you receive individual guidance about your own relevant precautions and contraindications for practice. You don't have to do all the activities in the book; trust yourself and engage with what seems helpful at a given time. Do not assume all the practices in the book will apply to everyone or that they will benefit you in the same way. Each reader has special requirements and it is important that you listen to your body and practice yoga with comfort. Move around, not through, pain. It is best to begin with the support of a yoga therapist who can help you with alignment, safety, and understanding the philosophy of yoga. This book does not replace medical or professional physical or mental health advice. Seek out and work with appropriate care providers. If you wish to connect with a yoga therapist, this book offers guidelines to find one.

Although it is written in sequence, you can move through the book however you are guided to do so. Jump around based on your own priorities, needs, and interests, or read it straight through. You may want to get a journal to record your personal thoughts, curiosities, and insights as you work through the book. As you begin to notice changes, do not abandon the practices and philosophies that are proving to be helpful. Continue to refer to this book and experiment with what is beneficial and what else could help.

A book is no substitute for professional training. It is no substitute for live instruction. It is no substitute for medical or mental healthcare. Please consider this book to be a starting point for a longer journey in this area that may take you many places or a supplement to what you are already doing. There are other research papers to read, other practices to try, and other teachers to seek out. This is simply a reflection of my years of experience witnessing profound changes for so many people, both quantitatively, and qualitatively. All of the stories are real. All of the practices are tried and true. All of the evidence is cautiously evaluated and presented with care. Practices in the book aim to shift lifestyle and perspective to reduce pain and gain greater meaning, purpose, and joy. We hope it serves you well.

Activity List

Chapter 1
Myths of Arthritis Quiz

Chapter 2
Breathing: Balancing the Autonomic Nervous System with Balanced Breath
Posture: Comfortable Ways to Sit

Chapter 3
Posture: Basic At-Home Yoga Practice
Relaxation: Body Scan
Breathing: Three-Part Breath

Chapter 5
Sense Your Energy Kosha
Relaxation: Heart Relaxation
Reflection: Reflection on Energy
*Breathing: Breath of Fire (*Kapalabhati Pranayama*)*
Posture: Sun Salutation Vinyasa *Supported by a Chair*

Chapter 6
Posture: Bed Yoga

Chapter 7
Concentration: Witnessing the Senses
Breathing: Breathing Practice for Inflammation: Sheetali
Concentration: Meditation Sampler

Chapter 8
Reflection: Gunas *Reflection Exercise*
Reflection: Self-Care through Established Practice
Relaxation: Awareness Relaxation
Breathing: Balancing with Nadi Sodhana *Breath*
Concentration: Pratyahara: *Calling the Senses Inward*
Reflection: Removing Obstacles to Practice
Posture: Terri's Strong Mountain

Chapter 9
Concentration Exercise: Discerning the Mind and Intellect
Posture: Subtle Asana *Practice*
Reflection: Living a Personal Intention

Chapter 10
Reflection: Arthritis and Your Dharma *(Purpose)*
Reflection: Rituals for Health
Posture: New York Yoga for Arthritis Sample Practice

Chapter 11
Posture, Relaxation, Breathing, Concentration: Joint Lubrication
Posture, Relaxation, Breathing, Concentration: Vinyasa: *Sun Salutation in a Chair*
Posture, Concentration: Vinyasa: *Moon Salutation (Chandra Namaskar)*
Posture, Relaxation: Restorative Sequence

Chapter 12

Posture, Relaxation, Breathing, Concentration: Yoga Practice Supported by a Chair

Posture, Relaxation, Breathing: Preventing and Managing Knee Arthritis

Posture, Relaxation, Breathing: Mini-Sequence: Finding Steadiness in Uncertainty

Posture: Mini-Sequence: Desk Yoga Poses

Posture: Mini-Sequence: Cultivating Inner Strength

Posture, Concentration: Mini-Sequence for Inner Peace

Chapter 13

Reflection: Your Healthcare Team

PART I

LIVING WITH ARTHRITIS

This part of the book offers you insight into many forms of arthritis and elucidates what it is like to live with this chronic disease. It also introduces yoga therapy and offers insight into how yoga is empirically linked to a range of benefits for arthritis. There is also a relationship between the medical model and yoga therapy. I introduce the *pancamaya kosha* (PMK) model of yoga, which, similar to the biopsychosocial-spiritual (BPSS) model of healthcare, views the whole person in order to affect the deepest levels of healing. Part I includes practices and personal reflections for readers living with arthritis and those who support them.

Chapter 1

WHAT IS YOGA THERAPY FOR ARTHRITIS?

This book is written for the average reader and designed for several distinct audiences, each of which may use it differently. People with arthritis and those who love them, health professionals, yoga teachers, and yoga therapists should all find something useful and inspiring in these pages. Many people with arthritis believe that yoga may not be for them. While certain types of yoga are not appropriate for people with pain, inflammation, or limited mobility, many styles of yoga have evidence of benefit for various arthritis symptoms. As you read this book, you have the chance to experiment with yoga practices. You will learn more about the different forms of arthritis and how symptoms affect many areas of life. Customizable solutions are here, too, in the form of easy-to-understand yoga theory and practice. This chapter focuses on demystifying and clarifying arthritis in its various forms and the impacts it has on the whole person living with it.

What Is Arthritis?

Even if you are not a medical or yoga professional, you probably know many people who have arthritis. In fact, while one in five adults in the United States is diagnosed with arthritis, it is suspected the actual rate is closer to one in three,[1] while one quarter of all Europeans have some form of arthritis.[2] There are some similarities in the effects of arthritis, for example pain, but there are also many differences. To know a few people with arthritis is not to know the disease itself. This is due to the many specific diagnoses that fall under the umbrella of "arthritis," as well as individual differences in the course, severity, and comorbidities of the disease.

"Arthritis" is a category of chronic conditions that includes over one hundred different diagnoses. When we break down the word "arthritis" we see it literally means inflamed (*itis*) joint (*arthro*). Common symptoms include joint pain, stiffness, and even deformity resulting from chronic inflammation and/or tissue damage. Tissues surrounding the joints are also affected, as are other connective tissues. Arthritis conditions can be autoimmune, and may also impact certain organ systems, muscular strength, and mood. Despite their different mechanisms, this book includes recommendations and explanations of yoga practices and philosophy that can have a beneficial impact on conditions as diverse as fibromyalgia, lupus, lyme disease, ankylosing spondylitis, psoriatic arthritis, polymyositis, and gout. While discussion throughout the book focuses on the two most common forms of arthritis, OA and RA, I encourage readers interested in related conditions to apply the information as warranted. I will speak in more detail about these other conditions later in this chapter.

Let me be sure to reiterate that I am not a medical doctor, merely a researcher sharing what I have learned in years of working exclusively with this population. The observations and practices in this book do not constitute medical advice. If you or your student/client is experiencing symptoms, seek proper medical attention—the earlier the better. It is never too early to mention a concern to your family doctor. It is better to be reassured about something minor than to delay adequate care.

MYTHS OF ARTHRITIS QUIZ

How well do you think you know arthritis? The following quiz is inspired by the pre-course work for Yoga for Arthritis trainees. Try the quiz below and test your arthritis awareness! It is a chance to find out more about arthritis and its treatment. Answer *true* or *false* to each statement:

QUIZ

1. If you develop arthritis, you should not exercise because it will further damage joints.

2. Arthritis affects only a few specific joints in the body.

3. The amount of time it takes to get a diagnosis and receive appropriate treatment is normally over a year.

4. If arthritis symptoms disappear, you have been cured.

5. RA affects men twice as often as women.

6. Gout is the mildest form of arthritis.

7. Arthritis medications are poison and should be avoided.

8. You must have swelling in at least three joints before arthritis can be diagnosed.

9. Arthritis is the leading cause of disability in the United States.

10. People with arthritis have some control over how they experience the disease. Everyday choices can be the difference between ability and disability.

ANSWERS

1. False: Exercise is an important healthy lifestyle practice. Sadly, the idea that it is better not to exercise is a common myth that may contribute to worsening arthritis symptoms over time. Exercise, such as daily yoga, walking, or swimming, helps keep joints moving, reduces pain, and strengthens muscles around the joints. Rest is also important for the joints affected by arthritis. Physical therapists can develop personal programs that balance exercise and rest. Exercise also helps keep weight under control, which reduces stress on the joints and may slow the progression of certain forms of arthritis.

2. False: Although arthritis is common in certain weight-bearing or often-used joints, it can affect almost any joint in the body.

3. True: It can take up to a year to get a proper diagnosis of systemic arthritis because many patients delay seeking care and it can take a while to eventually see a rheumatologist. It then often takes months to find an appropriate treatment regimen for systemic arthritis, which doesn't reflect poorly on the medical provider. Different treatments work for different patients. One size does not fit all.

4. False: There is no cure for arthritis, although medications and other treatments can ease the symptoms and slow the progression of the disease. Also, symptoms of arthritis may go away by themselves but then come back weeks, months, or years later.

5. False: RA is an autoimmune disease that affects women two to three times as often as men. Although RA most commonly begins when a person is in his or her 30s or 40s, the disease can strike at any age. No one knows why RA is more common among women; it is possible that the female hormone estrogen plays a role in disease development.

6. False: Gout is *not* the mildest form of arthritis; in fact, acute gout can be extremely painful. Gout is caused by a build-up of uric acid crystals in the joints and tissues. Swelling may cause the skin to pull tightly around the joint and make the area red or purple and very tender. In general, gout occurs most often in older men and affects the toes, ankles, elbows, wrists, and hands. Medicines can stop gout attacks, as well as prevent further attacks and damage to the joints. Reducing purines in the diet can also help.

7. False: While most medications do have some side effects, they can also literally save lives.

8. False: Swelling in just *one* joint is enough for an arthritis diagnosis. Other symptoms include morning stiffness, joint pain, or tenderness that is constant or comes and goes, and redness or warmth in a joint.

9. True: Despite how its impacts are often minimized, arthritis is often so severe it has become the number one cause of disability in the United States.

10. True: It is possible for people with arthritis to feel better. They have some control over how they experience the disease. Self-care is not an option; it is a necessity. Nutritional choices, activity levels, rest, and letting go of draining commitments are a few examples of how arthritis patients can promote wellbeing.

Now that you have tested your knowledge, continue reading for more interesting keys to understanding arthritis.

Who Gets Arthritis?

Anyone can get arthritis. With over 100 forms of the disease, I see clients from a range of demographics, lifestyles, and genetic histories. Arthritis and other rheumatic conditions have been the most common cause of disability among US adults for the past 15 years.[3] Almost 55 million Americans have been diagnosed by a doctor with some form of arthritis.[4] One study of over 600 individuals found that 14 per cent had undiagnosed inflammatory arthritis.[5] Additionally, arthritis prevalence is estimated to rise to 78 million by 2040, making up over 25 per cent of the adult population.[6] Once you begin to understand the risk factors for arthritis, such as obesity and inflammation, the reasons for this increase become clear.

While arthritis is not limited to older adults, the risk of arthritis increases with age. Of persons aged 65 or older in the US, almost half reported doctor-diagnosed arthritis,[7] and globally, that prevalence is up to 80 per cent for people over 65 in high-income countries.[8] As the world's population continues to age, it is estimated that degenerative joint disease disorders such as OA will impact at least 130 million individuals around the globe by the year 2050.[9] In fact, the prevalence of arthritis among individuals age 85 and older is expected to double in the next 20 years.[10]

Additionally, arthritis is more common among women than men and women tend to live longer than men do, so that in the next 20 years two-thirds of the arthritis population will be women.[11]

Physiology of Arthritis

Most forms of arthritis are marked by a deterioration of joint tissue. The specifics of how this happens differ by arthritis type. In OA, by far the most prevalent form, the cartilage that provides a smooth surface on the end of each bone is compromised. This is largely due to a mechanical process of wear-and-tear in which friction wears away at the cartilage. It is exacerbated by the pressure of excess weight, repetitive movements and/or prior injury. As nicks and cuts form in the cartilage surface, that deterioration accelerates. Osteophytes (bone spurs) also form in response to the friction, which add to the mechanical challenges. We now know that OA is not exclusively biomechanical, and that low-grade inflammatory processes also play a role. Further complicating matters, excess fat tissue is associated with increased systemic inflammation, thereby creating additional pressure on weight-bearing joints and also contributing to inflammation-related mechanisms.

Autoimmune forms of arthritis, such as RA, psoriatic arthritis, lupus, and ankylosing spondylitis, operate primarily through overactivation of the immune system, which preferentially targets joint tissue. In systemic arthritis, the whole body is affected; thus, other organs and body systems such as heart, lungs, kidneys, blood vessels, and skin may be compromised. Psoriatic arthritis affects a small percentage of people with the skin disease, psoriasis. It often affects the fingers and toes but can also affect tendon insertions into bones such as the Achilles tendon in the ankle. Lupus can affect organs, muscles, skin, or joints. It affects many more women than men and can vary greatly in severity. Ankylosing spondylitis exists in the spine and can result in loss of spinal mobility. It has a strong genetic component and often strikes young adults. In some of these systemic, autoimmune forms of arthritis, the process of the immune system attacking joint tissue starts with the synovial capsule, a membrane that surrounds synovial joints and contains the synovial fluid. Different types of cells that are part of the immune system are activated and create an inflammatory process that begins to deteriorate many aspects of joint tissue, including the cartilage.

There are some conditions in the umbrella of arthritis that do not directly impact joint tissue. An example is fibromyalgia, which is characterized by dysregulation of pain-processing in the central nervous system (brain and spinal cord). Because pain is prolific throughout the body, it was originally thought to be a musculoskeletal condition. When no visible pathology could be detected at the location of pain concerns, the condition and those who had it were generally not taken seriously. We now know that people with fibromyalgia and other pain syndromes have a very different experience of pain and sensation that can be helped by some of the same lifestyle changes that benefit people with arthritis. See Chapter 7 for a more in-depth discussion on this.

Gout is a common form of arthritis that is characterized by excessive uric acid build-up in joints, often including the big toe. Uric acid creates a crystalline structure in the joint that is extremely painful and can be addressed medically by reducing uric acid production or increasing its breakdown. Because uric acid is formed from the breakdown *purines*, a diet with reduced purines (found in red meat and beer, as well as other foods) may help to manage gout symptoms.

It is important to remember that these diagnostic categories are imperfect. In this book, I primarily talk about forms of arthritis that impact the joints, but many of the concepts and behaviors discussed will be relevant across all conditions. Each person is unique with a biology and psychology unlike anyone else. Some have said that rheumatology could have a different diagnosis for each person because these conditions behave differently in each person, and each person experiences and responds to them differently. The disease names give us a framework for talking about these conditions, acknowledging that generalizations often fail to adequately capture the experience of any single person. For this reason, I have also included many examples of personal stories that give you a glimpse into how this all happens outside of theory, in real life.

Osteoarthritis and Rheumatoid Arthritis

Let's compare the leading forms of arthritis: OA and RA. Most people who claim to "have arthritis" will likely have either OA or RA…and sometimes both!

The most common form of arthritis is OA, affecting over 30.8 million Americans.[12] It is estimated that by 2050, 130 million persons worldwide will suffer from OA, and 40 million of them will be severely disabled.[13] OA has been traditionally viewed as resulting from mechanical wear-and-tear in weight-bearing joints such as knees, hips, and spine, but can also affect non-weight bearing joints, such as hands, especially with overuse. Early in the disease, pain occurs after activity and rest brings relief; later on, pain occurs with very little movement, even during rest. OA is understood as a biomechanical process that impacts more than just the affected joints, but also includes some more widespread changes.[14] Mechanical wear is accompanied by decreased joint repair, contributing to joint damage.[15]

Although OA is primarily mechanically driven, there is also systemic inflammation in OA (although far less than found in RA). Scientists think that several factors may cause OA in different joints. OA in the hands or hips may run in families. OA in the knees and other weight-bearing joints is linked with being overweight and with biomechanical factors. Injuries or overuse may cause OA in joints such as knees, hips, or hands. Pain, the most common OA symptom, is affected by both psychological and biomechanical factors. Symptoms of OA can range from stiffness and mild pain that comes and goes to severe joint pain and even disability. Living with OA can be stressful because of symptoms and physical limitations.[16] Daily stresses can exacerbate pain, affect psychological health and contribute to disability.[17]

RA, on the other hand, is an inflammatory autoimmune condition, which not only leads to pain and swelling in the joints, but also results in loss of muscle tissue,[18] called "rheumatoid cachexia." Along with inactivity because of the symptoms (pain, swelling, fatigue, and more), this cachexia further reduces strength and physical functioning,[19] often hastening disability (see Chapters 4 and 6, where I talk more about the effects of muscle atrophy). RA can be highly debilitating. It causes damage to cartilage, tendons, ligaments, and bone. This damage can cause deformity and instability in the joints that leads to decreased range of motion. It can destroy joints and affect systems throughout the body. Signs of RA often include morning stiffness, swelling in three or more joints, swelling of the same joints on both sides of the body (both hands, for example), and bumps (or nodules) under the skin most commonly found near the elbow. Current medications alone are unlikely to eliminate the disability that happens with irreparable joint damage,[20] but early and aggressive medical management can greatly decrease an otherwise progressive and destructive disease course.

People with RA sometimes believe that OA is no big deal, when, in fact, there are some people with mild RA and some with severe OA. OA can be just as disabling in some cases, especially when multiple joints are involved. OA and RA are different diseases with different features. Note the following comparison in Table 1.1 to understand more about the similarities and differences between these two most common forms of arthritis.

Table 1.1: Side-by-Side Comparison of RA and OA

	Rheumatoid Arthritis	**Osteoarthritis**
Type of Disease	Autoimmune	Biomechanical (and more)
Symptoms	Joint pain Joint stiffness Decreased range of motion Systemic inflammation Fatigue Fever	Joint pain Joint stiffness Decreased range of motion Localized swelling
Location of Symptoms	Swelling in pairs—especially smaller joints, including wrists, knuckle joints of the hands, and feet	Usually weight-bearing joints (knees, hips, low back), neck, small finger joints, and big toe
Time of Day	Generally worse in the morning or after lack of activity	Tends to get worse throughout the day with activity
Age of Onset	Usually 30–50 years, though can occur at any age	Most commonly middle-aged and older people
Prevalence	1.5–3 million people in the US ≈ 1% of worldwide population	26 million people in the US 630 million worldwide

Medical Interventions for Arthritis

No matter which of the many forms of arthritis are at play, it is important to receive and follow clear medical advice. The main medical interventions are assistive devices (walkers, canes, splints, braces, etc.), medication, and surgery.

Assistive devices are products or equipment that help keep the body safe or perform certain actions. By helping to stabilize the body and aid movement, assistive devices offer a higher level of function. There is more opportunity to move, work, and fully participate in life. Tools like orthotics, electric can openers, or elevated toilet seats can improve quality of life for a person with chronic pain and limited mobility. While assistive devices provide relief, they do not address the root cause of the issue.

Medications are a key aspect of arthritis treatment, as they directly address inflammation and pain, among other symptoms and features of the disease. The kind of medication prescribed depends on the type of arthritis in question, as well as the specific needs of the person. Table 1.2 explores the most common types of medications prescribed for arthritis.

Medication is part of a personalized treatment regime. It is essential to take the medication as prescribed and communicate any side effects or concerns with your healthcare team. Do not alter the medication course on your own; rather, work with your doctor to adjust dosage and type of medication. Never stop taking any medication without discussing it with your prescribing doctor. Some medications are prescribed to be taken "as needed," which is sometimes written as PRN (*pro re nata*). This is generally true for pain medications that are bought over-the-counter (without prescription). While some medications are used only to manage symptoms, others are an important tool for preventing disease progression and keeping inflammation at bay. This depends on the specific diagnosis, as well as disease severity. If you notice changes in symptoms after incorporating yoga into your self-care routine, it is important to share that observation with a doctor and have a conversation about disease status and treatment options. It is critical to foster clear and open communication with the medical team through the inevitable fluctuations of rheumatic disease.

In some cases, doctors may recommend surgery. Surgery can provide relief of pain and improved quality of life. It may, however, put restrictions on future activity level and lifestyle. Surgery may not provide relief from back and sciatic pain, for example. It may give initial relief, but many patients find that over time their pain returns, sometimes worse than before. Surgery often damages surrounding tissues and may present unpredicted outcomes. Before attempting surgery, it is best to consider the lifespan of the surgical technique in addition to all potential management strategies, such as weight loss, strengthening surrounding tissues, and addressing pain. Anyone considering surgery should ask a doctor about all of the other potential options first, including fitness and learning to work with or around pain. If the choice is made to proceed with surgery, it is important to set a timeline with a doctor for preparation and recovery, ensuring full awareness about the risks and recovery process, and options to delay the surgery while other management strategies are pursued. On the flip side, it is important not to delay surgery unnecessarily. Oftentimes, patients tell me that they should have proceeded with surgery earlier for all the relief it brought, and it is important to maintain physical strength and fitness prior to surgery, which can be difficult if the arthritis is severely progressed.

Table 1.2 briefly describes the most commonly prescribed pharmaceuticals for various forms of arthritis. The chart includes type of medication, effects, and side effects. For all of these drug classes, it is important to consider potential drug-supplement interactions, which should be discussed with the prescribing provider.

Table 1.2: Most Commonly Prescribed Medications for Arthritis

Pharmaceutical	Intended Effects	Side Effects
Corticosteroids	Systemic anti-inflammatory effects in RA, psoriatic arthritis, and other inflammatory diseases	Cortisol is a hormone that regulates the body's stress response, so using corticosteroids for long periods may decrease the body's own cortisol and its protection against stress Some of these types of medications impact the immune system, which may increase susceptibility to infections Long-term use may cause bone thinning (osteoporosis), increase blood pressure (hypertension), and increase blood sugar (diabetes)
Non-Steroidal Anti-Inflammatory Medications (NSAIDS), including over-the-counter and prescription medications	Reduce pain Reduce inflammation Because they treat symptoms, they do not actually affect the disease, but they can help patients function in daily life	Long-term use may cause stomach-lining irritation (gastritis) and ulcerations May affect kidney function and blood pressure May increase risk of cardiovascular disease
Disease-Modifying Anti-Rheumatic Drug (DMARD) Various types available, often in combination with other pharmaceuticals	Decreases symptoms of RA Slows joint damage by reducing inflammation	Methotrexate, the most commonly used DMARD: Nausea, fatigue, headache Interferes with folic acid metabolism (recommended to supplement this vitamin, which may reduce other side effects, too) May impact liver function and blood counts as well as bone health Not recommended during pregnancy
Biological DMARDs Administered by injection	Decreases inflammation and symptoms of RA and other systemic, inflammatory, autoimmune conditions Reduced bone damage	Suppress the body's ability to fight infection Other side effects vary by drug class

Yoga as Non-Pharmacological Treatment

In addition to the medical interventions listed above, there are numerous complementary and integrative health (CIH) approaches that have been shown to help with the pain and inflammation of arthritis. Movement-based therapies such as yoga and physical therapy help by strengthening muscles, supporting joints, improving alignment, and releasing endorphins. Anti-inflammatory food choices and dietary supplements may reduce inflammation, soothe pain, and decrease insomnia. Mind-body approaches like meditation and relaxation found in yoga aid in reducing stress and pain levels. Physical manipulation like hands-on massage or osteopathic adjustments help mobilize tissues, decrease pain, and improve circulation. As I will discuss continually throughout this book, the best non-pharmacological interventions are the everyday lifestyle choices made by people with arthritis to support their own physical and mental wellbeing.

Yoga is not just one activity, but a whole lifestyle with practices that can serve someone with arthritis in its many forms and stages. In researching yoga for arthritis, I maintain a view of the totality of yoga and its impacts on the whole person, across all areas of life. When we teach yoga to people who have arthritis, we don't strive for a magical *asana* sequence that will address arthritis in a particular body part. Instead, we offer the various tools of yoga to the person living with arthritis. In other words, yoga is a holistic process, not a medicine cabinet. When we make the mistake of thinking about yoga as if it were physical therapy, we lose what makes yoga a unique therapeutic process. Physical therapy is beneficial and important; yoga is too, but largely via different mechanisms. While yoga can go hand-in-hand with modalities like physical therapy, it is a complementary process that aims to shift the experience of the body-mind.

Researchers, clinicians, yoga professionals, and yoga practitioners lose something when only considering an *asana* sequence and its effect on the joints. Instead, my focus is on getting the joint challenges out of the way—through support, use of props, compassion, and awareness—so that the whole of yoga can work its magic on the whole person: body, mind, and soul. While the typical treatment paradigm for arthritis and other chronic disease tends to limit itself to directly addressing physical limitations, symptoms, and progression, our model for wellness includes awareness, education, and growth. By viewing wellness as a whole-person experience, beyond simply the physical presentation of the disease, we are able to improve overall wellness no matter how much physical health deteriorates. We must remember that physical health, psychological state, level of independence, social relationships, personal beliefs, and lifestyle/environment all impact the overall health of a person.[21]

When people face arthritis, they are likely to also encounter some form of functional limitation/disability, physical symptoms such as pain and swelling, depression/anxiety, an unfamiliar level of reliance on others, and a change of roles—socially, occupationally, and domestically. Yoga provides a source of empowerment during these shifts in function and role by offering the kind of no-impact physical activity that is safe and effective for people with arthritis.[22] Yoga for Arthritis accommodates individual differences and encourages participants to explore their ever-changing needs and abilities in their own ways. Mindfulness, relaxation, and breathing exercises add an extra dimension to the process, allowing for deeper personal reflection and shifts in perspective that can dramatically improve health. Throughout this book, as I discuss how yoga therapy works with the many layers of a person, you will have many opportunities to learn about and explore the multidimensional benefits of yoga practice.

When we published the first study using the Yoga for Arthritis protocol in 2015,[23] it was the largest and most rigorous study of yoga for people with arthritis. We set out to compare the effects of yoga and usual care interventions on physical aspects Health-Related Quality of Life (HRQL) for people with RA and OA after eight weeks. We also explored potential mediators of that effect by assessing change in the markers of physical fitness, psychological functioning, and disease symptoms. In the end, we discovered that after eight weeks of twice-weekly yoga classes plus home practice once per week, there were statistically significant improvements for the yoga group compared to usual care. That said, there is no evidence that this is the best yoga program for people with arthritis. My background in Integral Yoga informed the research classes and they yielded statistically significant results. The Integral Yoga format has not been proven better or worse than any other style of yoga; no study has been done comparing it to another program a person with arthritis could do.

At the end of the eight-week study, flexibility, walk time, tender and swollen joints, positive and negative moods, depressive symptoms, and a global assessment all revealed significant changes. Self-reported change in physical health, perceived stress, pain, general health, physical roles and function, social function, and mental health were also significant. Furthermore, these changes persisted at the nine-month follow-up, and, anecdotally, many of the participants are still practicing yoga a decade later! Some of their stories are featured in this book.

During our research, we found evidence to support the notion that yoga is not perceived as accessible to everyone. Unfortunately, through turns in historical events that have been discussed in the social science literature, yoga in the West became a practice of young, thin, college-educated white women. Unfortunately, this leads many people to believe that yoga does not welcome them, or that they will not be able to do it. I believe that it is the responsibility of yoga professionals with a platform to communicate that union between mind and body is not reserved for one particular demographic. It is a birthright of being born with both mind and body. I hope this book will reach some people who might otherwise feel reluctant to try these practices. I hope it will encourage medical professionals to recommend yoga to their patients regardless of demographics. I hope it will better equip yoga professionals to serve those whom yoga's philosophy and practices have not already reached.

Yoga in Empirical Study

While evidence regarding the health effects of yoga has been collected and disseminated for many years, it was not always been done in the manner of modern scientific inquiry. Case reports in the modern medical literature date back almost one hundred years, but clinical trials are more recent. Early studies aimed to determine the safety and feasibility of yoga. In other words, is it safe and will people do it? Such studies had small sample sizes and small budgets and were often conducted as passion projects by researchers with other (more serious and reputable) scientific career trajectories.

Once the safety had been fairly well established in many different clinical populations, trials to determine efficacy were underway.[24] These studies were also relatively small and often contained only one arm, meaning that one group was recruited, received yoga, and was then assessed for changes. While this is a reasonable next step, it cannot be determined whether the measured changes were due to other factors, or due to the yoga. On order to determine that, researchers must include a comparison group to see if the same changes occur over time in the absence of yoga. Early comparison groups were usually "usual care" (standard medical care as usual) or a waitlist control, as was used in our first study 15 years ago.

Since yoga involves attention from a caring professional, it is ideal to have a comparison group with "equal attention" since we know that attention alone can foster health improvements. Such comparison groups might include an educational class, support group, or some form of exercise. The comparison group choice depends on the outcomes of the study, the population, and the study aims. Sometimes, a study will include more than two comparison groups and may look at yoga compared to an active control and compared to an inactive control (no intervention).

Once we know that yoga is associated with health changes beyond those derived from attention, we want to see how yoga compares to current best practices. Such studies are often called "non-inferiority" studies. They are not trying to show that yoga is better than other treatments, but just that it is another effective option for people who would prefer it. (To show that yoga is "superior" would require a much larger sample size and greater expense than simply showing non-inferiority.) Such a study was recently conducted for low back pain and showed that yoga therapy was not inferior to physical therapy.[25]

Ideally, we would then want to begin comparing different types of yoga practices to figure out what might be most effective for particular populations or to foster a certain outcome. We might compare a gentle yoga practice to an athletic yoga practice. We might compare poses with controlled breathing to poses without controlled breathing. We might compare meditation to chanting. Or we might look to see the differences between different frequencies or durations of yoga practice. This is the next step in yoga research and it has hardly begun. Until this type of research is conducted, it is difficult to say what practices might be most appropriate or most beneficial. Instead of direct evidence, we must rely on expert opinion, patient perspective, and traditional wisdom to inform the development of yoga programs.

Our research must be considered in the context of the overall trajectory of yoga research, which has increased exponentially in recent years (Figure 1.1).[26] Each research study must be considered for its methodological rigor, bearing both strengths and limitations. While our studies adhere to numerous standards, such as random assignment, blinded assessors, broad outcome measures, and racially diverse samples, we still faced limits such as small sample size, low generalizability, non-specific effects, dose distribution, and possible psychosocial ceiling effect. When you evaluate research on yoga for health—or any empirical study—be aware of design. There is always room for further research, building on the contributions of what came before. A research team I am a part of recently proposed an explanatory framework for yoga therapy, informed by ethical and philosophical perspectives.[27] We include four philosophical perspectives (phenomenology, eudamonia, virtue ethics, and first-person ethical inquiry) to provide a means of understanding how yogic practices, including lifestyle ideology, support an individual's transformative experience of illness, pain, or disability. I personally look forward to continuing to move yoga research toward greater rigor, transparency, and usefulness.

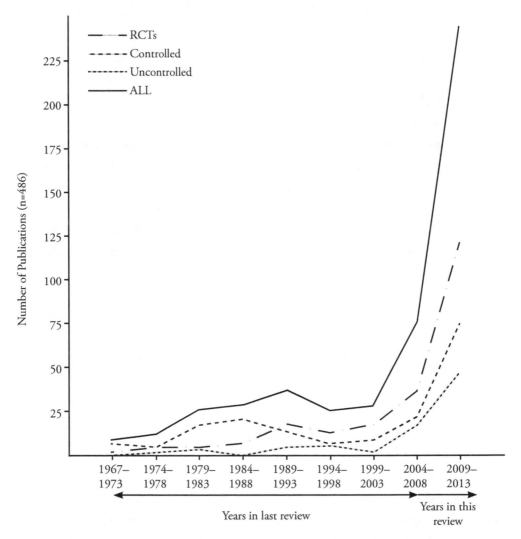

Figure 1.1: Trajectory of Yoga Research

Johns Hopkins Yoga for Arthritis Class

Our first study on the effects of yoga for people with arthritis was at Johns Hopkins Arthritis Center. We offered a 60-minute Integral-based yoga class twice per week for eight weeks and included instructions for weekly home practice. Each class took place in a hospital's fitness or recreation facility and followed the same format. I designed the yoga program with the support of the Johns Hopkins Arthritis Center faculty, starting with my training as an Integral Yoga teacher, and adapting the program to the study population. We agreed that a comprehensive yoga practice was warranted, including the elements of controlled breathing, meditation, mindfulness, physical postures, relaxation, chanting, and philosophy.

From a physical perspective, classes began with slow, gentle movements, and gradually progressed in difficulty. Standard yoga props were available (blocks, straps, blankets, chairs), and poses were modified based on individual needs and limitations. Participants were encouraged to try new skills, but to remain safe in their execution, refraining from doing movements that led to joint discomfort. New elements were added by building upon skills from prior classes. The intention was to provide a well-balanced class, including forward bends, backbends, twists, balances, standing, sitting, and lying-down postures, all with modifications for joints affected by arthritis, as described in the Appendix.

The home practice gradually built over the eight weeks from just a short meditation to an hour-long practice, in addition to supplemental readings about yoga practices and arthritis. We included the home practice so that participants could practice three times per week without having to travel to class so often. Additionally, we wanted to ensure that once the study was over, they would have the tools and confidence to continue practicing on their own.

The overall class structure was the same each week and followed a general arc that is common among many styles of yoga. Below is a detailed explanation of the class structure. Any researchers interested in replicating the study, utilizing the same protocol adapted to a different population, or collaborating on research in this area can contact me for a copy of the full protocol. While it is probably a slog to read any doctoral dissertation, this study was the subject of mine; for someone who is very interested in the research, I am happy to share that document also.

Classes began with five minutes of discussion facilitated by the teacher, based on homework from the previous class. This was either an article they had read or a yoga practice. Students had an opportunity to ask questions, share their experiences, and troubleshoot any challenges to home practice. For example, after a wall class, students were asked to try a Warrior Pose sequence at a wall in their homes. In discussion, it became clear that many homes do not have a stretch of empty wall and it was unrealistic to ask arthritis patients to remove art from the wall or start rearranging furniture for their yoga homework! They were, however, very creative in helping each other find solutions to challenges such as this, thereby overcoming barriers to practice.

Once participants had the chance to debrief, the class was guided to focus on their seated alignment. While a small percentage of students started out in a chair, everyone in the study was sitting on the floor by the end of the intervention. The decision to start in a chair was often due to fear of not being able to get back up afterward, but as they built strength and agility, this concern subsided. (See Chapter 10 for a related story.) Everyone in the study was able to get up and down from the floor safely with proper instruction. Whether seated in a chair or on the floor, many variations were used to ensure comfort and proper alignment to optimize spinal elongation and deep breathing. After attending to postural matters, students engaged in diaphragmatic breathing (see the first part of the three-part breath described in Chapter 3), mindfulness, and chanting. Benefits of these practices for mind and body were discussed.

I am often asked about chanting and there is some science to suggest its benefits. Additionally, it is, indeed, a component of yoga and therefore belongs in a comprehensive practice. In the Johns Hopkins study, we were able to chant the sound of Om without resistance from university administration and participants. We also chanted *om shanti* at the end of class and I explained the meaning of both chants. In some contexts, it is appropriate to change the chant from a Sanskrit word to a word that will be more accessible to the population, such as *Amen, Shalom*, or *Salaam*. In the replication of this study elsewhere, we were asked by the Institutional Review Board to exclude any chanting. In such a situation, I would generally encourage participants to audibly sigh like a long, slow, expressive letting-go. This can even be accompanied by the mouth sounds of *ah, oh*, or *mm*, thereby fostering the same resonance as the traditional chant.

After these initial centering practices, we moved into joint mobilization to lubricate the joints, and warm-up major muscle groups. This was done seated comfortably, then legs were extended, then students moved onto hands and knees (with props as needed) before coming to standing. Every major muscle group and every synovial joint was engaged in the warm-up, with coordination of breath and mindful awareness. Students were always encouraged to find their own version of the movements with many options offered, and it was delivered as a playful exploration. (A similar sequence can be found in the warm-up outlined in Chapter 11.) In other contexts, I have led similar mobilizing sequences in chairs or standing.

Once standing, students found Mountain Pose (*Tadasana*), which is a neutral standing pose with attention to alignment, mindfulness, and breath. This was followed by Sun Salutation, which was generally done with the support of a chair or with blocks for elevation. It can also be done at the wall, which accommodates a greater range of height and mobility. The Sun Salutation is a sequence that allows for fluid, full-body movement. It can lightly engage the cardiovascular system, which is important for a sedentary population that may be losing cardiovascular fitness from both deconditioning and disease processes. The Sun Salutation can be found in Chapter 11. A Sun Salutation tutorial and practice are also available on the Arthritis-Friendly Yoga DVD, which I created with the Arthritis Foundation.

The Sun Salutations were followed by standing postures that engaged strength, flexibility, and balance. Poses were used for their appropriateness for the population, their common use in general yoga classes (for sustainability of practice), and to ensure a comprehensive whole-body practice. I also explained the energetics of each pose (grounding, surrendering, heart-opening, energizing, etc.) and how it might be considered a metaphor for life with arthritis (see Terri's Strong Mountain in Chapter 8 for an example of this).

After standing poses, students returned to the floor for supine stretches, a mild inversion (hips above heart) and seated postures. These poses were held longer than standing postures and allowed students to stretch, cool down, find calm, and bring their awareness inward in preparation for deep relaxation. These poses were followed by a modified whole-body mudra (energetic seal) focused on gratitude toward body, self, and whatever else arises.

Deep relaxation was conducted in the style of Integral Yoga, starting with a tensing and releasing of all major body parts to foster release of muscle tension. This was followed by a mental scan of the body from toes to head to relax further. Attention was then brought to the breath to lengthen the exhale and engage relaxation of the nervous system. The mind was then brought into awareness to reduce fluctuations and foster stillness of mind. Next, students were encouraged to connect with a sense of peace residing within them. They remained in silent relaxation for several minutes.

Following relaxation, students returned to sitting to notice the effects of the practice. This was followed by a responsive peace chant (*Om Shanti*) and a short silent meditation. In meditation, students were encouraged to choose any focus for their attention, such as the breath, a word, image, or personal prayer. They were instructed that if the mind wandered from that focus, they should bring it back to the chosen focus with loving kindness. This instruction was provided to avoid self-judgment and an inner story related to the "success" or "failure" of the meditation. Becoming aware that the mind has wandered and returning it to focus is successful meditation. The effects of meditation were also mentioned.

Class concluded with a traditional bow of thanks between students and teacher. Students were then reminded of their homework to be completed before the next class (article or home practice) and students were afforded the opportunity to approach the teacher after class for personal questions, concerns, or updates. Any students who missed class unexpectedly were called to ensure that they were okay, remain engaged, and to suggest continued home practice before next class.

Is Yoga for Everyone? The Issue of Inclusion

While anyone who met the criteria for our research was welcome to participate, we know that not everyone feels welcome in the current culture of Western yoga. Arthritis does not discriminate and neither should yoga. Yoga should be accessible to anyone with a body and a mind. In our research at the Johns Hopkins Arthritis Center, we recruited a diverse sample of people with RA and OA for a randomized clinical trial studying the effects of yoga on quality of life and other outcomes. While approximately half of the participants who enrolled for the study were non-white minorities, race was the single greatest predictor of attrition (dropping out of the study). In most cases, participants dropped out of the study before classes even began.

While the prevalence of arthritis is slightly lower among African American and Hispanic people than among non-Hispanic white people in the US, the impact of arthritis in these groups is actually greater. The prevalence of activity limitation, work limitation, and joint pain are significantly higher among black and Hispanic people.[28] Minority ethnic persons with arthritis are more likely to delay joint replacement, and likely to have poorer health status both before and after surgery, including wellbeing, pain, and physical function.[29] In RA, disease activity, clinical outcomes, and remission rates differ between whites and minority groups.[30]

Racial and ethnic disparities in health and healthcare are well documented, and these patterns in arthritis are also reflected in other health conditions. They may be related to access to or use of health services, as well as language barriers and cultural differences. Willingness to report limitations, pain, variations in patterns of medication use, and approaches to pain management may also play a role. Additionally, the risk factors associated with arthritis, including obesity and manual labor, are higher in these populations. Life stressors may also partially account for racial/ethnic differences in disease activity among patients with autoimmune arthritis, such as RA. Because of these disparities in treatment and outcomes, minority persons with arthritis may stand to benefit most from non-pharmacological disease management strategies and self-care practices, such as yoga, to complement medical care.

It is possible that some of the explanation for minority attrition in our study was related to differences in socio-economic status and access to resources like transportation, childcare, and predictable work hours, which can impact study participation. I also considered, however, that yoga in the West is practiced mostly by young, thin, white, flexible, college-educated women. Given that I, the face of the research study, fit all of those categories, perhaps I was part of the problem. I was interested in finding ways to make yoga more accessible and acceptable to those who could benefit most.

As serendipity would have it, soon after that study ended, I was contacted by a researcher at the National Institutes of Health who was interested in the same problem. We wanted to know whether race/language/ethnic concordance improved acceptability of yoga among minorities with arthritis. In other words, are people more likely to practice yoga when the teacher looks and speaks like them? We worked with a large and very diverse research team (I was the only monolingual white person) and thought about all of the ways to make yoga more accessible. This impacted decisions like where and when to hold the classes, what the materials should look like and even the inclusion of family members. Much was learned during that study.[31] The process highlighted how easy it is for underserved minorities to be left out of the conversation and the solutions. Without effort towards inclusion, optimal health and healthcare will continue to serve those with the greatest access instead of those with the greatest need.

There has been some work done by the Arthritis Foundation to demonstrate that people with arthritis come in all shapes and sizes—they are all ages, all shades, all levels of ability.[32] Such a campaign aims to reduce biases and assumptions about people living with arthritis. Similarly, there is a movement called Accessible Yoga that aims to make yoga accessible to everyone, regardless of ability, age, size, or background.[33] Both of these campaigns are important for reducing disparities for underserved minorities living with arthritis. I am mindful to speak out about these concerns whenever I see people being excluded from representations of arthritis and of yoga.

Summary

Arthritis and the people affected by it are diverse. As arthritis rates continue to increase internationally, it becomes more important that there are a range of available interventions. Yoga, its philosophy and practices, offer important interventions. One of the intentions of this book is to create an inclusive framework of yoga that can be adapted both physically and philosophically. Use the aspects of this book that make sense for you. Those aspects that are not a fit for your lifestyle or professional practice can be left out. I do advocate that you understand yoga is a whole-person practice, not just a series of poses, just as arthritis is a whole-person disease. The following two chapters describe these concepts in greater detail.

Chapter 2

ARTHRITIS IS A WHOLE-PERSON DISEASE

How often do you apply the concept of body-mind-spirit health? Do you consider yourself and your patients/clients in relation to all areas of life? This book encourages you to consider the whole person. This is a means of seeing yourself and others not only as a body but also an energetic, emotional, reasoning, and spiritual being. This whole-person perspective is essential in arthritis management. Whether or not the arthritis is systemic, it is important to consider the impacts of disease on a person's overall physical, mental, and spiritual health. Arthritis impacts people on all of these levels by limiting movements, energy levels, relationships, careers, and even sense of self. This chapter gives you an overview of how arthritis affects the whole person.

Several whole-person models exist, each one addressing the individual as a multilayered being. Our bodies, breathing habits, energy levels, emotions, thoughts, beliefs, social engagement, lifestyle, interests, and aptitudes must all be considered. The whole-person models discussed in this book are the BPSS model from the modern medical perspective, the concept of HQRL that is often measured in empirical studies, and the PMK model from yoga, described in the following chapter. This chapter discusses the first two of these important frameworks for understanding the many ways that arthritis impacts people and how yoga therapy may be of benefit.

Arthritis as a Whole-Person Condition

Arthritis can impact all areas of life. People with every form of arthritis report poorer quality of life than those without.[34] This can be due to decreased physical function, emotional consequences, or a change in the roles they play. It may make people feel hesitant about participating in social activities, where they may feel incapable, embarrassed, or like they are slowing other people down.

It is clear through my research and personal experience with this population that arthritis impacts overall quality of life. Many people living with arthritis experience fatigue, trouble sleeping, depressive symptoms, and even social isolation. It is often accompanied by pain and can interfere with activities of daily living such as grocery shopping, walking the dog, or sitting at a desk.

These physical, emotional, and lifestyle features relate to one another. Because of the pain and fatigue caused by arthritis, it becomes challenging to perform all the tasks necessary for self-care and upholding relationships and work. In time, life narrows for a person with arthritis, as even completing the bare necessities can feel like a stretch. It is common for people to miss social engagements, thereby limiting the social network of support. Often, the mind resists the physical pain and people feel frustrated by their lack of control over the symptoms and impacts of the disease. Depression, anxiety, anger, and despair are common outgrowths. The physical symptoms, isolation, harmful thoughts, low emotions, and challenges associated with daily responsibilities makes arthritis a whole-person disease.

BREATHING: BALANCING THE AUTONOMIC NERVOUS SYSTEM WITH BALANCED BREATH

The nervous system is highly involved in the whole-person range of arthritis symptoms. The autonomic nervous system (ANS) has two branches: sympathetic nervous system (SNS, your "fight-flight-or-freeze" response) and parapsympathetic nervous system (PNS, your "rest-and-digest" response). The SNS responds to stress, whether real or perceived, by increasing the heart rate and blood pressure, releasing stress hormones, and sending more blood to the muscles instead of the digestive system. The PNS, on the other hand, allows the bodily systems to restore and has a soothing effect on the emotions. The overactive SNS leads to many stress-related mental and physical health problems. The overactive PNS may manifest as apathy and lethargy. It is beneficial for us to have balance in the nervous system: the PNS is active enough that we are uplifted and calm while the SNS is active enough that we are engaged in life.

This practice works well to balance the nervous system, mind, and emotions. It is commonly recommended by yoga therapists to cope with a variety of situations. I recommend that you repeat this and other practices throughout the book, familiarizing yourself so that you do not need to continually consult the instructions as you gradually make them a regular part of your routines. Try the balanced breath yourself or with clients and enjoy the effects!

1. Notice your breath. You don't have to change anything; simply witness its depth, rhythm, and presence. Similarly, tune in to the kinds of thoughts you are thinking and the range of emotions that are with you.

2. Count the length of each inhale and exhale. Allow the breath itself to find its own pace. If you are not accustomed to breathing exercises, it may speed up at first as the nervous system gets used to something new.

3. Allow each inhale and exhale to become a similar length. Eventually, your breathing may find an equalized inhale/exhale ratio. As you maintain an equal count, observe any shifts in what you are thinking and feeling. You may choose to extend each equal breath. Without being competitive, add a beat to the inhale/exhale count as it feels natural to do so. When you relax into that, you may add another beat if that feels available.

4. Breathe normally. Let go of your attempts to equalize and prolong the breath. Notice how you feel, what your thoughts are, and the way the breath moves without your direction.

You can use this practice at any time to help balance your mind, body, and nervous system. When we are more relaxed, we are more resilient to stress, our organs function better, and we experience less pain. When practiced without force, equal breath is an excellent tool to support nervous system balance. This, in turn, promotes a whole-person sense of balance.

A Common Path through Arthritis

Over the past 15 years, I have heard hundreds of arthritis "origin stories" that describe first signs and symptoms, how they progressed, when medical support was eventually sought, and how it was treated. Of course, as with everything in life, each of these stories is unique. There are, however, a few common themes that have emerged throughout the course of our Yoga for Arthritis studies.

OA almost always starts with dull joint pain. For younger folks, this occurrence is often a joint that has been previously injured, perhaps including surgery. It could also be a joint (or joints) that are overused repetitively. My grandmother was a knitting teacher who developed arthritis in her hands and fingers. Someone who does manual labor while kneeling might get arthritis in the knees. Usually it seems to begin slowly and progress gradually. The pain might start occurring only after long periods of use, such as long sessions of typing at a computer or walking all day. Over time, the pain starts after shorter periods of use and grows in intensity. I often see people stop an activity to hold or rub the affected joint(s) to bring some rest and comfort. Eventually, the pain might begin to feel ever-present, changing in intensity with the weather, the time of day, or activities. By then, most people have mentioned it to their family doctor or primary care provider (PCP). The PCP might observe the joints and tell the patient that it is likely arthritis, or that they could be getting arthritis. Some people just assume they have arthritis because they have joint pain, and perhaps they have relatives with OA. A diagnosis of OA, however, requires at least a radiograph (x-ray) of the joint to see how much space exists between the bones. This space tells us how much connective tissue has been degraded in the joint. The image might also show osteophytes (bone spurs) and other abnormalities in the joint structure. This is useful because it can allow a doctor to track the progression of the arthritis over time and it may inform choices about how/when to intervene.

Systemic forms of arthritis, like RA, tend to come on less gradually, progressing over weeks and months rather than years. They may start with one joint but eventually tend to involve multiple joints. A combination of symptoms often includes pain, stiffness, and swelling, perhaps with fatigue and even a low-grade fever. Symptoms may increase consistently or they may come and go in waves. Occasionally, the onset can be sudden and dramatic, like waking up one day with a knee the size of a grapefruit. As RA tends to start at a younger age, most people don't suspect arthritis. I've been surprised to hear that even in some families where rheumatic diseases are already present, it doesn't always lead to early diagnosis and treatment. Oftentimes people first go to their family doctor, sometimes after a long period of suffering with no care. The PCP may suspect an injury, which may be referred to an orthopedist or other specialist. I have heard many stories where a year went by between the first experience of symptoms and a diagnosis. It further complicates matters that arthritic conditions vary so much. Even once referred to rheumatology, it can take a bit of time to figure out exactly which disease it might be. However, there are also some cases where a single trip to the PCP results in an immediate referral to rheumatology and a quick diagnosis.

Once systemic arthritis is diagnosed, it can also take some time to find appropriate treatment. Often this starts with steroids to quickly address inflammation while the slower-acting medications take hold. The steroids are then often tapered to a lower dose or no dose. There can be a process of trial and error with the type of medication and the appropriate dose. This can be frustrating for patients and their families, but I think it is helpful to know that this is typical and eventually you will find something that works. In this process, it is so important to communicate openly with your doctor about what you are experiencing and for physicians to encourage this rapport. Consider the care to be a collaboration that requires patient input, feedback, and cooperation as you find effective treatment together.

Also know, and this is an important opportunity for some yoga philosophy, things will change. Yoga teaches us to accept the ever-changing nature of reality. In the case of arthritis, this means that whatever works may eventually stop working, perhaps temporarily and perhaps permanently. Symptoms may resolve and they may recur. Because of this, ongoing and trustworthy healthcare is critical to long-term arthritis management.

For any form of arthritis, the medical care doesn't happen in a vacuum. Lifestyle choices, like diet, physical activity, rest, stress management, and mindset, can have a major impact on how well the arthritis is managed. The tools of yoga offered in this book can help improve awareness about changes in the bodily experience that are key to disease management. Yoga also provides some specific techniques and lifestyle recommendations that may reduce symptoms and improve quality of life in every stage of an unpredictable chronic disease. The following story shows how a highly debilitated person can find profound transformation through yoga for arthritis.

Marina's Story

I first met Marina when she came to the Johns Hopkins Arthritis Center in desperation. She was not the typical person you would expect to see in a Yoga for

Arthritis class: early 20s, healthy looking, and apparently mobile. Nonetheless, at just 23 years old, she felt as though she might be 83.

Marina was in pain and suffering with RA. She had been diagnosed with RA at age 16. She was a serious ballet dancer at the time and the symptoms of RA interfered with her dancing—an important part of her identity and future plans. In an era before widespread use of blogs and social media, there was not a rich network of support for young people with arthritis and Marina felt very much alone. She wished that she could find just one other person like her. She had a very grim outlook of her future and was even told by a medical doctor that she would be crippled by age 25. Marina did not want to believe this and was angry for having been given this sentence. Yet in some ways she took it to heart.

Marina's symptoms, as for many with RA, responded almost immediately to stressful situations. There was no separating the events in life, or her emotions, from the symptoms of the disease. Her parents were aware of this and when a beloved grandparent passed away, her father took her out to a restaurant for dinner as a way to soften the difficult news. Marina's joints swelled so responsively that her father had to carry his fully grown daughter out of the restaurant.

When Marina went to college, she knew that her RA medication could not be mixed with alcohol. She was resentful of being denied what she saw as a typical college experience and she chose the alcohol over the medication. She wanted to participate in college life the way those around her were doing. She felt distanced from her body and wondered why her body hated her so much. She certainly did not feel compelled to care for or nurture her body, which lately had given her nothing but pain and hardship.

By the time she got to Johns Hopkins, she was in search of anything that might bring her some relief. In fact, she moved to Baltimore after seeing that Johns Hopkins was rated #1 in rheumatology by U.S. News and World Report. Her years of medical non-compliance had taken a toll on her joints and she yearned for a glimmer of hope that something could be different. And that is exactly what she found. The rheumatologist she saw assured her that he could help her to improve. Fortunately, she believed him.

While at the Arthritis Center for a visit, Marina saw a flyer posted on a bulletin board in the lobby. It described our research study looking at the effects of yoga for people with arthritis. Since she had been a dancer, but didn't feel able to dance, she thought this might be something she could try. Her new rheumatologist agreed that this would be a good fit and she joined one of the first cohorts of our study.

The body awareness Marina established through her dance training was immediately evident in her *asana* practice. She quickly picked up alignment cues and was willing to try poses that challenged her fitness and helped her reconnect to her body. She was the youngest participant in her particular cohort and, despite the challenges of her RA, was the most mobile and agile in the group. We found modifications to address the limitations from deformity in some of her joints, particularly wrists and ankles. She excelled in the physical practice, remained engaged in all aspects of the class, and appeared to be enjoying the program.

Several weeks into the session, the class was practicing a small bridge pose. Some just lifted an inch off the floor, others used the wide side of a block under the sacrum for support, or rolled up and down through the spine. Marina, on the other hand, was lifting herself so high up in the bridge that both shoulder blades were off the floor. Seeing her willingness, I asked Marina if she would like to try moving into a full wheel pose (she didn't have any RA involvement in her spine) and she was reluctant. We quickly moved on. But two classes later, she was willing to try. I offered support under her ribcage and pelvis as she slowly lifted from bridge to wheel. I didn't realize it at the time, but this was a pivotal moment for Marina. She was supporting her own weight in a movement that was familiar to her—from before her disease! In particular, she was supporting her weight on a joint (her wrist) that had previously been an impediment even in routine activities. She had an epiphany that her body *could*, in fact, support her—that she and her body could be on the same team and could work together toward a goal.

No longer at odds with her body, Marina decided to take better care of it so that they could work together. She became compliant with medications and started eating a healthier diet. She even started running half-marathons with the close supervision of her rheumatologist, and has been able to minimize the severity and dose of her medications. She certainly still experiences stress and challenges, including periods of debilitating symptoms. Unlike many women with RA who go into remission during pregnancy, Marina's symptoms worsened. If pregnancy is stressful, having two babies just a year apart (while working full time) is even more so. However, Marina manages her stress and the challenges in her life very differently now. She has learned to walk away from situations, people, and responsibilities that drain her and to focus her energy on what nourishes her. She makes different choices, both big and small, and she notices how those choices make her feel. That, in itself, is a yoga practice.

Marina was speaking to a group of yoga therapy students and was asked what she does to manage disease flares. In describing how she lays in bed for long periods, awake but without thought, she realized that she is meditating. Sometimes Marina goes to yoga classes (though she reports that many yoga teachers are not as understanding as she'd like) and sometimes she practices at home. She also incorporates breath awareness into her daily life. I would suggest, though, that yoga is not just something she does with regularity, but it is a way that she relates to her body and her disease. In a very literal sense, Marina is experiencing a kind of *union* that has fostered greater self-care, greater awareness of her body's changing needs, greater compassion for herself. As such, she serves as a model for other young people with RA. Marina has become the very example she wished she'd had so many years ago.

Marina's story reminds us that arthritis can affect anyone, at any age, no matter their lifestyle. It is inspirational to consider how she found a way back to loving herself and her body through yoga. The yoga practice not only improved her physical health but also impacted her state of mind and perspective on life and her disease. She is not alone in this transformational journey. As you continue to read the book, you will see the many ways yoga can improve all realms of life for people living with arthritis.

How to Get Up from the Floor

In Yoga for Arthritis, we teach several different ways to get up from the floor. One way is to start on hands and knees (Table Pose), with any props that may be helpful. This can include a folded blanket under the knees for cushioning or perhaps a wedge under the palms to support the wrists. The toes are tucked under in order to press up into Downward Dog. From here, you can slowly walk the hands toward the feet or the feet toward the hands into Standing Forward Fold. Bend deeply at the knees, place hands on thighs for support, and lengthen the spine. Press into the hands to come up with a long spine and find Mountain Pose.

For those who are unable to tuck the toes under or press up into Downward Dog, the following option might work better. Begin on hands on knees with a blanket beneath the knees for comfort. You might want to have a chair in front of you with the seat facing toward you for support. Bring one leg forward with the foot flat on the floor, so that the foot is beneath the knee and the thigh is parallel to the ground. If using a chair, ensure it is set on a yoga mat to avoid slipping. Place hands on the seat of the chair to assist you. Press the hands into the seat of the chair to bring the other foot flat on the floor and then press up to standing with a long spine to find Mountain Pose. To perform this option without the chair, engage the abdominals and press hands off the front thigh, straightening the front knee to bring the other foot flat on the floor and come to standing in Mountain Pose.

A third option requires more arm strength but works well for those who have too much knee pain to be in Table Pose, even with cushioning. Sitting on the floor, arrange a stack of blankets, pillows, or a bolster behind you. A second stack should be a bit higher, perhaps two bolsters, depending on their thickness. Behind the second stack is a chair with the seat facing toward you. Place a hand (palm or fist) on each side of your hips and on an exhale press into the floor with the hands so you can lift your seat up onto the bolster (or other cushion) behind you. From there, bring the hands to the second stack and repeat so that you are sitting on the stack. Then bring the hands to the chair and press yourself up to sitting on it. Sit to the front of the chair, press the hands into the thighs, lean slightly forward, and on an exhale press up to standing.

The reverse of these three methods can be used to transition from standing to seated.

POSTURE: COMFORTABLE WAYS TO SIT

Throughout this book, you will encounter numerous practices and recommended ways of incorporating yoga into the average lifestyle. For many people with arthritis, even the simple act of sitting—something most of us take for granted and a position we assume for hours each day—can feel nearly impossible. The following offers some alternative ways to approach sitting so that it can be safe and comfortable for a body with arthritis. Change position as often as necessary and trust that sitting for longer periods will become more tolerable with time as strength and flexibility improve. Do your best to sit up on the sitz bones, which are the pointy bones you can feel through the flesh of your buttocks when you are sitting.

For many people with arthritis, Easy Pose (*Sukhasana*) isn't so easy. The typical cross-legged posture of yoga is more comfortable when the hips are elevated. Sit on folded blankets, a cushion, or bolster to raise the hips, which takes the pressure off the hips and low back (Figure 2.1). Sit as high as necessary to allow a natural curve of the lumbar spine. Each knee can rest on the opposite lower leg or one leg can be in front of the other. It is also an option to place blocks or rolled blankets beneath the knees to support the sensitive joints. Half or Full Lotus postures, which may come to mind as the classic seated yoga pose, are not appropriate or necessary.

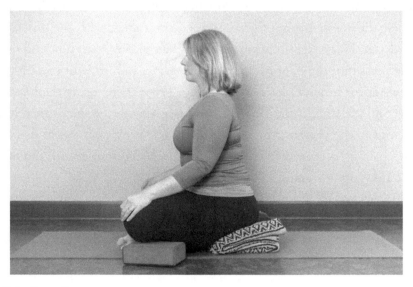

Figure 2.1: Easy Pose

Modified *Dandasana*, Staff Pose, is a similar option where you straighten one or both legs out in front rather than exerting the added pressure on the knees that a cross-legged position entails (Figure 2.2). Most people will want to sit up on something in this pose also to reduce pressure on the low back. In this case, I also suggest a rolled blanket or block beneath the extended knees to provide support.

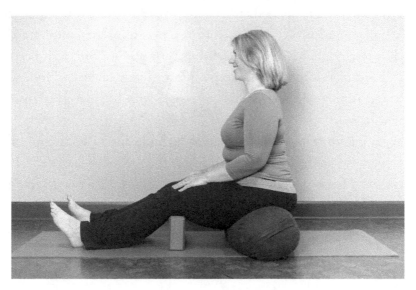

Figure 2.2: Staff Pose

Supported Hero Pose (*Virasana*) has the legs folded under the hips. It is most comfortable if there is a folded blanket beneath the knees to cushion them from the ground; keep the ankles under the hips to be sure not to twist the knees. Straddle a block or bolster so that your hips and torso are supported and the full body's weight is not pressing down into the knees (Figure 2.3). Placing a blanket over the block or a stacking a second bolster under the torso, can increase comfort. This pose can be gentler on the hips, but might be too intense for some people with knee pain.

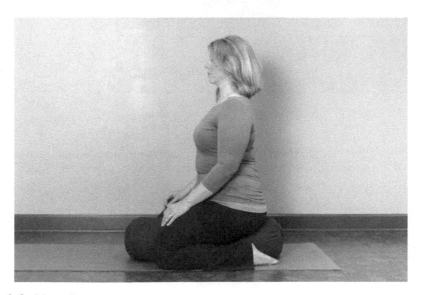

Figure 2.3: Hero Pose

Sitting on the floor trains the body to get up and down, thereby building strength, flexibility, and confidence. This mobility practice translates into practical life activities like reaching into low kitchen cabinets or playing with kids on the floor. It is even a life skill that can help to keep someone living safely and independently into older age. It may not be accessible to people with high levels of disability or who are new to yoga.

While getting up from the floor may be difficult due to joint pain or muscle weakness, there are strategies that can help to make it more feasible.[35] Putting a folded blanket or bolster below the knee can help, as can using a helping hand or seat of a chair for assistance.

Until one is ready to experiment with sitting on the floor, a chair is a suitable alternative. It is still yoga even if we are sitting in a chair. It is most important in all seated poses to sit up tall and lengthen the spine (Figure 2.4). A padded chair or blanket on the chair seat may be more comfortable.

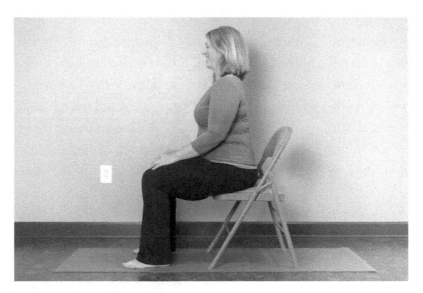

Figure 2.4: Seated in a Chair

In each of these variations, comfort is key. I will discuss different kinds of pain and discomfort in the section "Noticing Sensations and Responding to Pain" in Chapter 4, to help you or your clients discern when to back away from pain and how to remain safe and healthy in yoga practice. Experiment with these various ways of sitting as a way to learn more about your body and how it feels.

The Bio-Psycho-Social-Spiritual Model

For much of modern history, medicine has been dominated by the biomedical model, which looks at the biological causes and effects of illness. The biomed-ical model typically does not emphasize psychological, social, or spiritual aspects of health. In recent decades, however, there has been more consideration of the whole person, including the ways in which psychological and social factors are causally linked with biological health and how illness impacts mental, social, and spiritual health.

The biopsychosocial (BPS) model of health was proposed in 1977 by Dr. George Engel.[36] It is a theoretical framework that guides research and more comprehensive clinical care. A decade later, some scientists proposed that spirituality also be considered. Using broad measures in health assessment is aligned with the BPSS model. This model recognizes that a person is more than a body and that all of these components (biology, psychology, sociology, and spirituality) can impact health *and* can impact each other! Our systems don't exist in isolated silos, but as parts of an integrated whole. For example, the biology of arthritis (joint damage) can impact psychology (depression) and sociology (isolation) and spirituality (hopelessness). And the reverse is also true. A sense of connectedness can improve mood, relationships, and even pain.[37] The BPSS model acknowledges the interrelatedness of aspects of human life and health, no longer reducing humans to a body with interrelated functioning parts. It has always been important in my research to consider broad measures of health that are aligned with a BPSS approach.

Health-Related Quality of Life

There are lots of ways to measure health. Some of those measurements are objective, like blood pressure, and some are subjective, like pain. If we want to get an understanding of how someone feels, we use subjective measurements. Some people are healthy by standard measurements but don't feel good. The opposite is also true—some people don't have very good health but somehow manage to feel great! An example of this is knee OA. Research has shown that pain is not a strong predictor of tissue damage.[38] This means that someone can have a lot of pain with mild arthritis or very little pain with more advanced arthritis. Because of this, we need both kinds of measurements to really address each person's needs without making false assumptions.

Medical doctors rely heavily on objective measures, like a blood test to gauge inflammation. These measures are important for determining the severity of someone's disease, how quickly it is progressing, what treatments are appropriate, and whether those treatments are working. However, they only provide part of the picture. Doctors now routinely ask about pain, which is a step in the right direction, but even that can be a limited consideration of whole-person health.

Subjective measurements, like fatigue, consider the patient's point of view and how well one is living with disease, not just the nature of the disease itself; they also help us consider side effects or unanticipated challenges related to a treatment. We can compare the effects of a treatment for different people in different situations when we measure many aspects of someone's wellbeing. As a researcher who ultimately hopes to help people live more joyfully, the subjective measurements—the ones that measure how someone feels—are the focus of my work.

There are countless ways to measure the patient's perspective. These are called "patient-reported outcomes," or PROs, and fortunately, they are increasingly considered in medical care. One way to get a general idea of the patient's experience with a disease is to measure HRQL. It includes many areas of life that can be impacted by a disease like arthritis, including physical health, mental health, emotional health, and social health. When we used HRQL measures to assess the effects of an eight-week yoga intervention, we found improvements in pain, general health, energy, physical roles, physical function, social function, and mental health, with most of those changes persisting nine months later.

As healthcare evolves, it also follows a whole-person approach, emphasizing comprehensive multi-level models, ranging from individual cellular processes to broad environmental characteristics. Using validated instruments to assess HRQL, we are able to measure how whole-person interventions such as yoga therapy improve both the objective and subjective experience of the condition.

Summary

Arthritis impacts many areas of life. It is not just a joint disease or condition of the connective tissue affecting the physical body. Investigation and intervention should include the body as well as the whole, complex, unique person living with arthritis. The repercussions of arthritis, like most chronic diseases, can include functional limitations, physical symptoms, depression, and other mental health issues, low energy, social isolation, financial distress, loss of independence, and unexpected shifts in relationships and career. Arthritis is the leading cause of disability in the United States; it can lead to shocking limitations and influence upon everyday life.

Established measures of HRQL can assess how well one is living with the many BPSS aspects of arthritis.

Arthritis is both impacted by and has impacts upon all areas of life. Similarly, yoga is a whole-person practice which influences the body, energy, mental, emotional, social, and spiritual realms. The breathing exercises and postures, like some of those found in this chapter, and other traditional yoga teachings, help regulate the physiology, balance emotions, improve thought patterns, and bring a sense of spiritual connection. The focus of the next chapter is on how yoga touches many areas of life and health.

Chapter 3

YOGA IS A WHOLE-PERSON PRACTICE

Yoga, an ancient body-mind-spirit practice, continues to gain popularity—even within the scientific community. A few decades ago, yoga in the West was known and practiced only within a particular subculture. These days, people of all ages and from all walks of life enjoy the benefits of this whole-person practice. While yoga is now more widespread, the average person may not view it as accessible. Many stereotypes exist around who can and does practice yoga. As you continue reading, you will learn more about the kinds of yoga that are considered safest and most accessible, in addition to how you can find the type that is best for people with arthritis. For now, let us review yoga more generally.

What Is Yoga?

Yoga is a collection of ancient philosophies and practices originating in India. "*Yoga,*" a word from the ancient language Sanskrit, literally means "union" or "yoking."

This expresses its ultimate intention of joining the mind and body or the individual with the whole. The physical aspects of yoga, such as postures, breath work, and relaxation, were originally intended to prepare the body for seated meditation, an important spiritual practice in many cultures. Although its roots are in ancient philosophy, yoga's physical postures have become a common mind-body activity in modern Western society over the past few decades. Many people narrowly think of yoga as simply physical activity that helps with stress management, but the totality of yoga is much broader.

Even though calming the mind-body for overall wellbeing and connection may be the ultimate intent of yoga, the primary focus of yoga classes is often on strengthening, balancing, and stretching. While yoga may bring benefits similar to other forms of exercise, it is more than a physical activity, including such practices as controlled breathing, relaxation, cultivation of body awareness, nutritional choices, study of ancient texts, chanting, mindfulness, self-reflection, acts of service, moral living, and meditation. Different teachers emphasize different aspects; with just a few phone calls and simple questions, you can create a list of appropriate teachers for referral or inter-professional collaboration. If you are a yoga professional, be sure to introduce yourself to local healthcare practitioners and let them know the empirical benefits of your services. If you are a person living with arthritis, call ahead and ask what classes might be appropriate for you.

The Eight Limbs of Yoga

Throughout this book, I will be talking about the eight limbs of yoga. These limbs are practiced in concert; they are not necessarily sequential stepping stones. In fact, the more integrated we become in the subtler limbs of meditation and union with the self, the more important the early ethical limbs and external practices become. The first three limbs are the ethics of yoga or *yamas* (restraints) and *niyamas* (observances), followed by the physical practices of yoga (*asanas*). Directing the life force through breathing exercises (*pranayama*) is the bridge to the subtler limbs. The final four limbs are mastering the senses to quiet the mind (*pratyahara*), concentration or single-pointed focus (*dharana*), the altered state(s) of meditation (*dhyana*), and the supreme awareness or union with the Self (*samadhi*). This book offers you many opportunities to practice them, gradually gaining a more secure pathway to conscious awareness and the peaceful, higher perspective of *samadhi*.

What Is Yoga Therapy?

Yoga therapy is a profession that applies the tools of yoga to help address individual health concerns and foster a shift toward greater wellness. Yoga therapy considers the whole person, their individual challenges and abilities, as well as their concerns and goals. Instead of offering the same practices to everyone, yoga therapy customizes a plan of care, recommending specific (and often modified) yoga practices and philosophical applications as tools for self-care. While individual yoga therapists have been practicing around the globe for many years, it is in the last decade that standards have been developed for the training and credentialing of yoga therapists worldwide. As yoga therapy has become credentialed and professionalized, there has been greater integration of yoga therapists into healthcare settings, such as hospitals, senior care facilities, integrative health practices, and clinics. Yoga in these settings is being adapted for diverse patient populations. It is offered to people in hospital beds and wheelchairs, from pediatrics to geriatrics.

Unfortunately, the distinction between yoga classes for high levels of fitness and yoga therapy for help with managing chronic conditions remains unclear to the general population and even amongst many healthcare providers. While some of the research findings on yoga have been widely disseminated, the details about their highly adapted practices have not. Individuals with limited mobility sometimes seek local yoga classes, only to find that they are not accessible and may even exacerbate symptoms. One woman with arthritis was even told by her doctor—who practiced yoga himself—that yoga would not be safe. If his exposure to yoga was vigorous and athletic, it may very well be inaccessible to his patients. However, the tools of yoga are many, and anyone with a body and mind can bring them into union. Anyone can work toward greater mindfulness in the moment, contentment, and non-harming.

It is the role of yoga therapists to meet clients where they are, and to focus on the goals that are important to each client, while also recognizing potential areas for growth and greater wellness. While the ultimate aim of yoga may be union with the true self, the means to that end will be different for each individual; it might be a reduction in physical pain, improved stress management, or greater acceptance of current circumstances. Often, the intentions of yoga therapy change over the course of care, many times moving from gross, or obvious, to subtle. You see an example of this in the eight limbs of yoga described above. Yoga also provides a model of perceiving the whole person in view of this gross-to-subtle shift: the PMK model.

Yogic View of the Whole Person

Yoga has a system of understanding the whole person called the PMK model. This view perceives each person as five layers of being, moving from the most to least perceptible. The outermost layer is physical. Within that exists the energy/breath, then mental/emotional, wisdom, and ultimately bliss/spiritual connection. You may recognize this whole-person approach from the BPSS model described in the previous chapter, which acknowledges the layers of influence on a person's wellbeing (Figure 3.1). Yoga offers us a means of connecting to and balancing each layer and this balance can be assessed via HRQL measures, discussed previously.

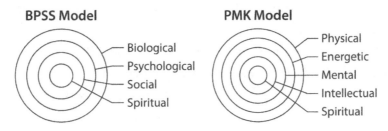

Figure 3.1: BPSS and PMK Models

The physical layer is the most obvious. We can connect to the body, or physical self, through movement, relaxation, or a simple body scan. Within the body is the energy layer, and that is mobilized via the breath. The simplest way to tune into this layer is by noticing the flow of breath within the body. You may also try the Sense Your Energy *Kosha* in Chapter 5. As we continue through the *koshas*, we move into more subtle realms.

Within the breath exists the mind, or sense impressions and emotions. You can understand this as your thoughts and the interpretations of your sensory organs. This layer changes quickly (just notice how many thoughts you have in the course of one minute), but you can calm it by bringing awareness to your thoughts and feelings without judging them or by endeavoring to focus on one piece of sensory input.

More subtle than the mind is the wisdom layer, which contains not only the peaceful knowing of the "true self," but also our strongly held core beliefs. Unlike the mind, the wisdom layer is slow to change. You can get a sense of this level of being by acknowledging the underlying pattern in your more quickly moving thoughts. For example, thoughts about your upcoming plans, staining the deck, and your partnership may all hold a sense of time pressure, preoccupation with cleanliness, or enthusiasm about the outdoors. The themes that exist within the thoughts reveal the contents of our wisdom layer.

The wisdom layer is the closest to spirit and, despite whatever beliefs may exist there, still leads us to insights about our spiritual selves. Yoga does not define spirit, nor is it a religion. It simply acknowledges that there is a spiritual dimension to our existence. You can connect to this innermost layer through the things that allow the deepest relaxation or that bring you the greatest aliveness. What are you passionate about? What have you enjoyed since you were a child? When have you felt a pervasive sense of wellbeing? These inklings are connections to your spirit layer.

Whether considering yourself or your patients/clients, it is important to remember the whole person: body, energy, mind, intellect, and spirit. HRQL considers many aspects of existence as being important to health and the function of all the levels. Each layer of being described in the BPSS and PMK models influences the other—the layers do not function independently. For example, when the physical body experiences pain, it impacts emotional wellbeing and energy levels. Conversely, when we feel more stressful emotions, it can exacerbate arthritis symptoms and even facilitate flares in autoimmune arthritis.

Each of the five layers described in the PMK model gives us insight into important aspects of our being and lifestyle. It is possible to connect to each layer through various yoga practices such as postures, breathing, chanting, and meditation. Arthritis affects all levels of the self and yoga can help to improve quality of life through all layers of the self.

Yoga Benefits a Whole Person with Arthritis

When you think of yoga for arthritis, it is important to factor in the full breadth and depth of yoga. Yoga is more than physical postures. It encompasses an entire philosophy of human life, including a range of ideas and practices for many layers of being. In addition to physical benefits such as pain relief, physical stability, and muscular strength, yoga can improve stamina and energy, calm the mind, and balance emotions.

Beyond the benefits of increased physical activity, yoga emphasizes the acceptance of limitations. It increases body awareness and the potential need for accommodating changes in physical function. For example, arthritis requires ongoing monitoring of functional abilities and requires continual adjustment of activities, rest, and mental/physical demand. Yoga also promotes lifestyle balance, emphasizing relaxation training, stress reduction, and a positive outlook. Yoga's combined mind-body approach therefore has the potential to confer psychological benefits that lead to improvements in quality of life for those suffering with arthritis. Thus, in persons with arthritis, yoga may help to maintain or improve physical and psychological health.

The breathing practices of yoga may be useful for balancing energy levels and the nervous system. This can shift the experience of pain and stress in people with arthritis. Even when the physical practice is not appropriate due to the disease progression, the breathing practices remain available to people with arthritis.

In the more subtle layers of the mind and intellect, yoga's philosophical approaches and mindfulness/meditation practices continue to bring balance and whole-person health. The chronic pain associated with arthritis has an effect on the anatomical brain. However, meditation and mindfulness practices do, too! The meaning attributed to the pain in addition to the quality of other thoughts changes the way one lives with pain and can even alter the structure of the brain. Meditation and mindfulness empower people living with arthritis to choose their responses to the disease and its symptoms. As perspectives shift, it is possible to attribute meaning to and even gratitude for the lessons and changes that arthritis brings.

Yoga is not something that has to be practiced at a dedicated time for a solid hour or so. While time "on the mat" can be excellent, it is not the only way to experience yoga, nor is it the most practical for everyone, especially with arthritis. I like to think about how yoga practices can be sprinkled throughout the day. This might mean standing differently in the grocery line, breathing deeply while doing the dishes, relaxing the body at bedtime, or avoiding distraction at mealtime. In fact, the ultimate goal is to live in a state of yoga all of the time; this vitalizes the most subtle, spiritual, layer of the whole person.

Ultimately, while yoga offers a set of practices, it is less an activity than a way of being. As you think about a yoga practice for yourself or someone else, keep an open-mind about what that might look like, both in terms of how it fits a particular body, and also how it fits into a particular life. A whole-person approach to yoga lifestyle means incorporating it into everyday moments in a personally meaningful and beneficial way.

Yoga's Ethics

According to the PMK model, yoga views everyone as existing in five realms, thus acknowledging that everything we do affects everything else. There are ten fundamental ethical observances listed in the 2500-year-old work *The Yoga Sutras* ("Threads of Union"), which help keep us in balance through all five layers of being. These are the first two limbs mentioned earlier in this chapter. The first five ethics are a code of behavior, inviting us to refrain from harm. The next five are recommendations for inner peace and clarity. You will find that many of these concepts echo other ethical traditions around the world and are somewhat universal across time and culture.

The first five ethics are called *yamas*, or restraints. First and foremost, we restrain harmful actions and thoughts toward ourselves and others (*ahimsa*). The second ethic, *satya* is a truthful, objective perspective and honest way of life. *Asteya* means "non-stealing" and this third moral principle has us remembering not to take more than is freely given. *Brahmacharya*, the fourth *yama*, can be understood as "right use of energy" and will be discussed at length in later chapters. The fifth and final restraint, *aparigraha*, translates as "non-grasping." It supports peace of mind and limits the waste of physical or mental resources on wishing and wanting.

As we learn to restrain what causes harm, we also observe and uplift our habitual ways of thinking and feeling (*niyama*). *Sauca*, translated as "purity" or "cleansing," is the first *niyama* teaching the cultivation of health through the whole person. This includes lifestyle choices such as rest, nutrition, exercise, and friendships, as well as state of mind. The second ethical observance is contentment (*samtosa*), practicing peace of mind regardless of current circumstances. *Tapas*—translated as discipline, austerity, or effort—balances contentment: once we accept reality as it is, we can take clear, measured action in the direction of our best life. Self-study (*svadhyaya*) and surrender (*ishvara pranidhana*) are the final two ethical principles.

There are many opportunities to apply these ethical principles to life with arthritis. They allow people with arthritis to think differently about how to live with the challenges of symptoms and disease. There are many opportunities to avoid harm, be it through honesty with oneself about what is happening in the body and the best response, not wasting energy on unnecessary tasks, not stealing health or peace of mind, and not grasping for a different state or situation than the current reality. Cultivating health and contentment are disciplines in action, and, as we study ourselves, we learn to accept what truly is, surrendering to the reality of the condition while more firmly gaining a relationship with the truth of our being.

While I have seen all kinds of profound changes in the way people live with arthritis, I believe none have been more profound than when the philosophy is taken to heart and informs perspective. When infused in daily thought patterns, these concepts steady any ship and allow people with arthritis to weather any storm…although regular yoga practice also has a tendency to improve the skies for smoother sailing in general.

The ethical principles of yoga offer depths of peace and purpose that are possible in each day. These five restraints—non-harm, truthfulness, right use of energy, non-stealing, and non-grasping—combine with the five observances—purity, contentment, effort, self-study, and surrender—to support a whole-person approach to life and wellbeing.

A Quick Word on Safety

The following are the main things to keep in mind for ensuring safety in the physical practices of yoga. Remember that it is important to consider the whole person practicing yoga. We offer more specific precautions and recommendations in Chapter 4 and the Appendix.

First, if you are a person with arthritis, check with your healthcare team to get clearance to begin a new activity and discuss potential concerns. If you are a medical provider, you may provide patients with specific precautions; however, as we reiterate throughout this book, some form of yoga is appropriate for anyone with arthritis, even in cases of extensive physical disability.

It is best to begin practice with the guidance of a qualified professional, either an experienced yoga teacher or yoga therapist. For arthritis patients, emphasis on stretching and strength, posture, balance, and the ability to adjust pace and intensity are important components of a safe exercise program, all of which yoga encompasses. People with arthritis learn to listen to the body and mind so that they know the limits and work within them. Sometimes emotions or uncomfortable thoughts will arise. This is common and so is processing them with a mental health provider. Above all else, trust and accept whatever comes up, including discomforts that ask for adaptations to the postures.

While this book offers a lot of suggestions for how poses can be modified, the intention is to find safe, comfortable ways for people with arthritis to experience yoga. There are numerous ways to experience any given pose. I do not to prescribe arthritis treatment in the form of yoga poses. The goal is to make the postures, breath work, relaxation, and mental approaches possible, so the full experience of yoga can come through safely and effectively.

POSTURE: BASIC AT-HOME YOGA PRACTICE

Right now, you can begin a simple yoga routine at home. You don't need much space. Keep the movements slow and gentle. While a small amount of discomfort can be part of any new activity, do not do anything strenuous or painful, especially anything that increases joint pain.

Stay focused on the sensations and your thoughts as you perform the postures. Yoga works on all levels of your being, including emotions and beliefs. The simplest way to remain present with your whole experience is to continually bring the attention back to the breath. We will begin the following practice by observing your breath. Intend to learn about your body, breath, and mind as you go through the entire practice:

1. Bring your attention to the way you are inhaling and exhaling. Notice the muscles, tissues, and bones that move as you breathe. You may observe that some breaths are different durations and depths than others. Notice this with acceptance and non-judgment; without trying to change anything, just observe.

2. After a comfortable period of time, stand up if you aren't already standing and notice *how* you are standing. Experiment with finding a place where you feel strong and balanced. Rock slightly back and forth, side to side, and settle in the place where you feel even. Is anything different from how you usually stand? Step your feet wider apart and repeat this step. Notice the alignment of the whole body from feet to crown of head. How do you feel in your body right now? Just witness.

3. Ensure that your feet are comfortably wide apart. Let your arms hang relaxed at your sides. Find length in your spine, creating space between the vertebrae and begin to slowly rotate your spine left and right, small and subtle. Be sure to stay upright and keep the movements slow so that you can observe the details of your experience and make safe movement choices. Imagine small rotation through the entire length of the spine:

tailbone, sacrum, lower, middle, and upper back. Notice how you are breathing as you move.

4. Breathe in and raise your arms overhead or to whatever height is comfortable for you. Do this slowly so that you can experience what happens in your shoulders. Breathe out and rotate your wrists in one direction; breathe in and rotate them in the other direction. Breathe out, relax the wrists and elbows, and pay attention to how you lower your arms. Notice what happens with your body, breath, and thoughts at the end of the posture.

5. Breathe out and bend your knees slightly, keeping your weight towards your heels. Walk your hands down your thighs to begin a forward bend with a nice long spine. You might want to hold on to a countertop or the back of a stable chair as you come forward. Notice how the muscles around your midsection support your spine and keep your back strong, even as it stretches. If it feels comfortable, the head may bow gently forward as you hold for a breath or two. Exhale to come up slowly with a long spine, staying strong, and allowing your hands to help as they walk up the thighs.

6. Inhale and bring your arms to the sides with palms up if it feels okay for you. Fell an opening across the front of your upper torso. Acknowledge any changes in sensation, breath, and thoughts as you transition through the poses. You may shift your weight towards your toes. Exhale to lower arms and return to a simple standing position and observe your body, breath, and mind.

7. Inhale your right arm up to wherever it feels comfortable and imagine creating space between all the joints in the right side of your body: ankles, knees, hips, shoulders, jaw, and even the spaces between the ribs. Exhale to come to center then repeat on the same side two more times. Repeat on the left. What is the same/different on each side? Do different thoughts come up? How is your breathing?

8. Pick something pleasant nearby, like a view out the window, art, or a plant. Let your eyes relax as you look at it, deepening your breath and appreciating the beauty of what you are seeing. Tell your thoughts to enjoy it. Let your breath deepen and feel your eyes and the muscles throughout your body relax.

As you can see from this brief exercise, a yoga practice can be gentle and accessible. A few movements, performed with awareness and integrated with the breath, are all it takes. Carry inspiration from this simple practice and bring more yoga into your life!

RELAXATION: BODY SCAN

Even though relaxation is a natural, healthy condition for the body, most of us need to retrain our minds and nervous systems in order to relax. Our body and mind are evolutionarily primed to be diligent about possible harms and sometimes err on the side of overreacting. The ethics of yoga support us in living with a more relaxed state of mind and body. In yoga classes, some form of guided relaxation is almost always present. The following relaxation practice makes you more aware of your body and how your mind can help bring you a sense of relaxation.

The steps below guide you through a deeper bodily awareness. As you continue scanning the body, understand that some parts of you will draw more of your attention than others. It will be easier to feel some places than others, whether because of comfort, discomfort, or a simple habit of attention. One of the benefits of this body scan practice is that you get to pay attention to parts of you that you might not otherwise notice. With repeated practice, you will learn about where different sensations tend to appear and will even gain skill in relaxing certain areas for greater comfort. Remember, there is enough space in you for both pain and pleasure. Being human means experiencing both, in varying degrees and with much impermanence:

1. Start in a position that is comfortable for you. This may be lying down in bed, propped up on the couch, sitting restfully with the head supported or any other position where your muscles do not have to work. You will be in this position for five to fifteen minutes.

2. Notice what you are feeling in your hands. Is it easy to relax your hands? Is there pain anywhere? Comfort? What happens when your hands start to relax? How do you know they are more relaxed?

3. Carry the awareness through the body in a systematic fashion. Shift your perceptions from your hands to your wrists and lower arms, feeling them relax, then on to your elbows and upper arms. What is it like to relax the shoulders, neck, and jaw? How does relaxation appear on your face? Can you feel your forehead, eyes, cheeks, and lips relaxing?

4. Continue sending the relaxed awareness down your chest and abdomen, back and spine, and all the muscles, bones, and organs of those regions. Acknowledge the places of comfort and discomfort without getting distracted by a story of your experience or wishing things were different. All you have to do is observe what is there now.

5. Send your attention through your pelvis. Can you relax the deeper muscles of the pelvic and hip region? Feel your thighs and knees, lower legs and ankles relaxing. Enjoy the relaxed sense as it moves through the small muscles and joints of the feet and toes.

6. After scanning the whole body you may wish to repeat the scan again, pick one area to rest your focus or simply imagine your entire body relaxing as a unified whole.

7. You can perform this body scan relaxation every day to get to know your patterns of tension/relaxation and pain/comfort. The more adept you become at scanning your body, the easier it is to apply this practice anywhere you happen to be, whenever you need to relax.

BREATHING: THREE-PART BREATH

The full, three-part breath is a foundational breathing practice in yoga. This method is taught in most styles of yoga because it recruits the entire breathing apparatus and offers a complete, healthy breath. I will discuss more about the relationship between breath and health later in this book.

The three-part breath explores using the primary breathing apparatus: lungs, respiratory diaphragm, abdomen, intercostal muscles, sternum, and clavicles. As you practice making your breath more complete, you may even notice how the back, pelvis, and, indeed, the whole body can be involved in the process. You can actually perceive the PMK model in action as you practice this method. As you become comfortable with the three-part breath, notice its effect on your mood or thoughts. Often, people will report that their thoughts slow down or seem more organized and emotions come into balance.

Begin by bringing yourself into a comfortable seated position like one of those described in the previous chapter. Close the eyes and bring your focus inward. Lengthen the spine, creating space between the vertebrae from the tailbone to the top of the head while allowing the natural curve of the back. Notice any places of tension or holding in the body and allow them to release and soften. Focus on the breath, breathing deeply into the abdomen.

You may put a hand on the abdomen to make sure it moves out on the inhale and back in on the exhale. This may feel strange if you have not been breathing this way for many years. We sometimes forget how to breathe properly as adults; however, if you watch a baby breathe you will see that the belly expands on the inhale and draws in on the exhale. This belly breath, the first part of the three-part breath, reduces stress, and gives us greater lung capacity. It even tones the abdominal muscles as they expand and contract with each breath.

Wrap the hands around the lower ribs, spanning as much of the ribcage as possible. Continue with the abdominal breath and build the inhale into the ribs, as well. Feel the ribs flare out to the sides and even to the back as the intercostal muscles, between the ribs, expand with each inhale. Every time you exhale, feel the ribs knit toward one another again as the lungs contract and expel the air. Each inhale the abdomen rises, and ribs expand to the sides and back; each exhale, the ribs come together and the abdomen lowers into the body as the diaphragm curves back under the ribcage.

The third part of the three-part breath happens in the upper chest. Most shallow breathers keep the action of the breath in the upper chest and that can be stressful for several body systems. When layered with the other two parts of the breath, chest expansion completes a healthy, relaxing breath. Bring a hand to the chest, feeling sternum and collar bones. Continue filling the lower two parts of the breath as you have been, then allow the breath to fill all the way into the upper chest. The sternum will rise slightly and the collar bones may seem to spread. When you exhale, let the breath flow out of the upper chest, ribcage, and finally abdomen. When you inhale, breath to the belly, ribs, then chest. Continue filling and emptying the lungs in this way for ten more rounds.

This breathing practice is appropriate for almost anyone, at any time of day. By recruiting the entire breathing apparatus, the body receives more oxygen which, in turn, promotes its relaxation and regenerative processes. Simply by bringing more attention to a complete breath, you are creating greater health.

The *Ayurvedic* Point of View: Yoga's Sister Science

There is an entire science related to yoga, known as *Ayurveda* (from the Sanskrit *ayus*, "life" and *veda*, "science"). While much of this book focuses on yoga lifestyle and practice, it is helpful to also understand yoga's "sister science" *Ayurveda*. Like yoga, *Ayurveda* arose from the Vedic tradition and developed in India as a health science. *Ayurveda* is a holistic medical system that, like yoga, takes the entire person, lifestyle, and external factors into account. While yoga's primary focus was historically on attaining transcendent bliss and Divine connection, *Ayurveda*'s intention was to remove disease from people's bodies and minds. Some yoga therapists also have training in *Ayurveda* and use the tools of this sister science to guide lifestyle recommendations and selection of yoga practices.

A concept inherent to *Ayurveda* that is also often considered in yoga therapy is the notion of an underlying constitutional profile that impacts tendencies and challenges for the body-mind. Each individual is considered to have some varying combination of three constitutional aspects of *doshas* that can be considered in supporting better balance in life and health. While most people are thought to have a primary *dosha* and perhaps a second more dominant *dosha*, others seem to have a more even distribution of the three. There is nothing inherently positive or negative about a particular *dosha* profile. Ill health arises when any of them are out of balance. It is important to note that imbalances do not always arise in the primary *dosha*. You may also notice that Western society tends to value the characteristics of some *doshas* over others, but all are important and useful when well balanced and harnessed effectively. Below is a further explanation of each.

Vata energy reflects the qualities of air and ether (space). Dominant *vata* energy is associated with creativity, excitability, and quick changes in energy and mood. *Vata* predominant types are often quick-learning, but also forgetful and perhaps impulsive. They tend to be thin with dry skin and cold extremities and a tendency toward pain conditions.

Pitta energy reflects fire and water. *Pitta* types are often strong in body and mind, articulate and strong leaders. They may be very focused, confident, and even aggressive. They are sometimes passionate and competitive, but may become easily irritated. They tend to have a medium build, dislike heat, and are prone to inflammation.

Kapha energy reflects the qualities of water and earth. *Kapha* predominant energy is associated with a relaxed pace, loyalty, and steadiness. *Kapha* types tend to be slower learning but remember well and act deliberately, but also tend to hold onto things. They tend to have sturdy larger bodies, experience low mood, and sluggish digestion.

Characteristics of each of the *doshas* can be associated with arthritis (such as pain, inflammation, overweight), and arthritis can impact someone with any *dosha* profile. There may be a greater likelihood of some forms of arthritis being associated with particular *dosha* prominence, and I have some thoughts on this matter, but it has not been well studied by Western medical research. Additionally, *dosha* energies may shift and change over the course of an individual's lifetime. If you are interested in learning more about your *dosha* profile and how your choices may impact their expression, consider consulting with a fully licensed *Ayurvedic* professional.

Summary

Yoga is a whole-person practice and any of its components can start a cascade toward whole-person healing. Just as we learned in childhood how all bones of the body are connected, so, too, are all layers of the self. A shift toward balance in one area (for example, breath) can facilitate changes in other areas (for example, mood). Because yoga includes a variety of practices that impact different aspects of the self (physical postures, breathing practices, relaxation, meditation, etc.), there can be greater opportunity for whole-person healing. Imagine a long row of dominos being hit on one end, and then consider what would happen if the dominos were toppled in various places simultaneously. While it is possible to experience whole-person healing from a unidimensional practice, yoga's holistic approach is particularly well-suited to foster profound and observable changes in all areas of life. Yoga is for everyone. The next chapter gives you/your clients more safety tips, practices, research, and motivation.

Chapter 4

YOGA, THE PHYSICAL BODY, AND ARTHRITIS (*ANNAMAYA KOSHA*)

Arthritis affects the body in more ways that simply through joint inflammation. This chapter explores the broader physical impacts of arthritis and explains the ways in which yoga can support physical health. For example, there is an interesting relationship between body weight and arthritis, not only for the joint tissue, but throughout body systems. Hormones, mood, and digestion are all affected by both obesity and yoga. The field of medicine, which is primarily focused on the biological aspects of health, is moving toward more acceptance and inclusion of whole-person approaches such as yoga therapy. Yoga practices such as postures, movements, and breathwork can be used safely by anyone, as long as the approach is appropriately individualized. This chapter touches on all of these points as we discuss the role of yoga therapy in arthritis and healthcare, emphasizing safety and self-care.

The Paradox of Arthritis and Physical Activity

There used to be concern that exercise might increase inflammation and exacerbate arthritis pain; however, regular physical activity is now recommended as part of comprehensive arthritis treatment.[39] Although vigorous exercise is often intolerable and may not be recommended for many persons with arthritis, some form of movement activity is important to maintain health. The American College of Rheumatology (ACR), Osteoarthritis Research Society International (OARSI),[40] and the Ottawa Panel[41] note that stretching and strengthening exercises, such as those performed in yoga, can improve endurance and overall condition while helping to preserve physical abilities. These are useful skills when combating the fatigue and pain that often come with arthritis. When people maintain exercise regimes, they manage their arthritis symptoms better or experience them less. Yoga, when practiced appropriately, can be an excellent healthy movement practice for people with arthritis.

When someone with arthritis or other rheumatic conditions is new to yoga, it is ideal to work one-on-one or in a small group with a yoga therapist or teacher who specializes in joint conditions or has significant training and experience with this population. If that is not available, a gentle or beginner class may be suitable, especially if the teacher is aware of the condition and feels comfortable providing the individualized attention and recommendations that may be needed. It is not ideal to begin a yoga practice in a large class, with an inexperienced instructor, or with a DVD that cannot provide individual guidance and feedback. As a student gains confidence with how to modify the practice safely and appropriately, yoga can be done in a variety of settings.

Because yoga practice has so many variations and can be easily individualized, it is a great way for people with arthritis to access the known benefits of exercise in arthritis management. While there may be modifications and assistive props needed, once the proper orientation to safety and moderation is introduced, yoga is convenient and affordable to practice at home, without the need for expensive equipment or access to specific facilities. It is important to remember that yoga means union, and unlike some other physical activities, it requires complete focus and presence in the moment. The mindfulness of yoga is partly responsible for its health benefits and is also critical for ensuring safety in the practice.

Yoga practice helps preserve mobility,[42] reduce arthritis symptoms,[43] and prevent or address common comorbidities such as cardiovascular disease,[44] hypertension,[45] and obesity.[46] Holding poses builds strength by engaging muscles in isometric contraction.[47] Moving joints through their full range of motion increases flexibility,[48] while standing poses promote balance by strengthening stabilizing muscles and improving proprioception to reduce falls.[49] Thus, yoga incorporates several elements of exercise that may be beneficial for arthritis. Additionally, stress management techniques are recommended to help cope with the challenges of chronic illness and prevent a cycle of psychological stress, inflammation, and immune dysregulation.[50] Moreover, yoga's slow and non-competitive nature is fitting with a disease that may potentially increase in physical limitations over time. Yoga teaches self-acceptance and a truthful, non-harming approach to movement choices and other lifestyle decisions so that people may remain active and healthy for many years.

Arthritis, Obesity, and Yoga

Inactivity, and the resulting obesity, play a role in arthritis. There is likely to be a cyclical relationship between overweight and sedentary lifestyle, which can make arthritis worse. The fatigue and immobility that often accompany arthritis contribute to this cycle. "If you don't use it, you lose it" is a valid truth in this situation. In fact, as cachexia, or muscle wasting, progresses, there is not only a continual loss of strength and function, as well as increased inflammation, but also an increased risk of mortality. Overweight adults report doctor-diagnosed arthritis more often than adults with a lower body mass index (BMI). The rate of arthritis among obese adults is twice as high as the rate among adults with a normal BMI.[51] Increased body weight means more pressure and friction on weight-bearing joints, which are common sites for OA. Because arthritis is more common among older adults and those with a higher BMI, chronic diseases of aging and obesity, such as heart disease and diabetes, are more prevalent among those with arthritis.

Poor physical activity can lead to the onset and progression of arthritis.[52] Because of injury risk, the more sedentary lifestyle in our modern society (cars, convenient appliances, elevators, desk jobs, screen time, etc.) combined with the "weekend-warrior" mentality towards exercise may be a recipe for arthritis. Furthermore, even healthy individuals struggle with long-term exercise maintenance, let alone someone coping with pain and tiredness, with attrition (quitting) generally approaching 50 per cent after six months.[53] Another factor in the relationship between obesity and sedentary lifestyle is that body fat is not inert tissue; instead, it could actually be thought of as an endocrine gland. More body fat is associated with changes in hunger and satiety hormones (the ones that tell us when we're hungry and when we're full) and increased systemic inflammation.[54] So, obesity makes it more difficult to maintain a healthy weight, more difficult to prevent arthritis, and more difficult to manage it once it occurs.

A sedentary lifestyle is a risk factor for the onset and progression of arthritis, but arthritis is associated with movement limitations. Twenty-four million US adults have both doctor-diagnosed arthritis and arthritis-attributable activity limitations.[55] The pain and potential joint destruction associated with arthritis translate into difficulty with a wide range of activities that limit the ability to work, live independently, or participate in leisure activities, thus affecting quality of life. The reduced levels of activity from pain and swelling contribute to a loss of functional ability. Because of this, people with arthritis are at greater risk for comorbidities (other conditions) related to lack of physical activity. In fact, adults with arthritis are about 2.5 times more likely to have two or more falls and suffer a fall injury in the past 12 months compared with adults without arthritis.[56] Those who have fallen are more likely to be cautious about activity and this fear of falling decreases activities (and therefore fitness and physical health) even further.

According to the Centers for Disease Control and Prevention, approximately one-third of adults who are also clinically obese also have arthritis,[57] and the rate of overweight and obesity has continued to increase, while morbid obesity has gone up over 60 per cent.[58] Obese adults with arthritis are almost twice as likely to be physically inactive as obese adults without arthritis.[59] Obesity and arthritis worsen each other—the more overweight a person is, the more stress on the joints and painful the activity; thus, one may avoid exercise and gain more weight, which, in turn, exacerbates the arthritis. Every pound of excess weight exerts four additional pounds of pressure on the knees.[60] Obesity, then, is a risk factor for OA. Additionally, it is associated with a more rapid progression of arthritis and worsening symptoms. Fat tissue creates and releases chemicals that promote inflammation. Due to increased inflammation, physical limitations, mental health issues such as depression, and a sedentary lifestyle, obesity and arthritis often occur together.

The benefits of weight loss on arthritic symptoms are many. Losing fat tissue means losing inflammatory tissue. For every ten pounds lost, there is a decrease in a whopping forty pounds of pressure on the knee joints. In a study conducted with my mentor at Johns Hopkins, we found that just 5–10 per cent reduction in body weight was associated with pain improvements similar to those with medication.[61] And as discussed earlier, less weight means greater energy, and because exercise is often a social activity, it improves quality of life in many other areas, too. Yoga offers potentially life-saving options to offset cachexia. Customizable movements in the form of *asana* help maintain or build muscle tissue. There are examples of people in this book who were so debilitated they could barely move but with patience, gentleness, and persistence were able to gradually build strength, reduce inflammation and fatigue, and support their bodies and minds in gaining health through yoga.

While it is generally challenging to start any new habit (think of New Year's resolutions), especially a physically active one, the best approach for safety and sustainability is to adhere to moderate-intensity exercise, taking it easy when in a flare and exploring greater challenges during spans of health. However, since this moderate approach is still not attained by the majority of those with arthritis, it is important to find suitable classes and learn about how to stay safe. Yoga is associated with weight loss—and not for the reasons most people think! Although most styles of yoga are not high in caloric expenditure, it does increase muscle strength, which, in turn, improves metabolic rate. Furthermore, the mindfulness practice cultivated in yoga also happens off the mat; therefore people are more likely to eat with appetite awareness, choosing appropriate amounts of food, and even making healthier choices as they notice the effects of food selection on overall sense of wellbeing. Yoga improves stress response, thereby reducing cortisol levels, and regulating leptin and ghrelin, all of which are hormones linked to stress-related weight gain.

Yoga impacts emotions and lifestyle, too. It is common to feel flooded by feelings and even laugh or cry during yoga practice. It is recommended that people seek support from a counsellor, yoga therapist, or trusted friend to help process these thoughts and emotions. It is also possible that the inward exploration of yoga practice may lead to changes in other areas of life. Many times these are positive changes (healthier eating, better sleep, etc.), but sometimes the practice of yoga leads people with arthritis to bigger life questions related to meaning, purpose, relationship, and roles. These big questions often ultimately lead to positive changes, but the process can be challenging. If you or your students/clients are struggling with these types of questions, it may be appropriate to seek professional support in the form of a counselor, social worker, religious guide, or medical doctor, depending on the concern. People living with chronic conditions often tell me about their "network of support," including a variety of professionals from various arenas to be called on as-needed. Find someone you can trust and consider them to be an important resource when challenges arise.

Yoga may be uniquely suited to a long-term practice because it can be continuously modified as needed, the benefits are so broad, and it engages the participant fully. In fact, our research shows that after eight weeks of practice, the benefits are sustained nine months later,[62] and, anecdotally, many people who participated in our yoga research program ten years ago are still practicing yoga regularly today and reaping the benefits of long-term practice.

Since weight loss slows the progression of arthritic symptoms and yoga is associated with weight loss, even in populations that require a greater modification of poses or more gentle postures,[63] yoga is an excellent intervention to slow the progression of arthritis.

Does the Gut Impact Arthritis Symptoms?

People actually have many more bacterial cells than they do human cells. As such, we are more of an ecosystem than an individual. While we think of these bacterial cells as separate from us, they closely interact with our own cells and tissues. Perhaps the place in the body where this most apparent is in the digestive tract, which has the greatest proportion of bacterial cells and a large presence of the immune system. The digestive tract is like an open tube with bacteria of all kinds flourishing throughout, and immune cells are active throughout the lining of that system.

Behavioral and lifestyle factors change the bacterial composition of the gut, and this affects immune function. These may include diet, supplements, medication use, stress, and even sleep.

Changes in the gut microbiome (bacteria living in the gut) are more easily and logically implicated in autoimmune conditions such as colitis and inflammatory bowel disease, there are also links between certain strains of gut bacteria and forms of arthritis such as juvenile idiopathic arthritis (JIA)[64] and psoriatic arthritis.[65]

Another mechanism by which the gut microbiome impacts arthritis and related conditions is through something called the *gut-brain axis*. Much as the nervous system involves bidirectional communication between the body periphery and the brain, the gut-brain axis characterizes signaling between the brain and digestive tract. This communication helps to foster homeostasis in multiple systems, including hormones, immune function, and nervous system. The balance of gut microbes may alter the function of this system via the nerve and immune cell activity.[66] Changes in gut immunity can then alter gut-microbe diversity. This is further complicated by the effect of stress hormones on neurons that change characteristics of the intestinal lining and therefore bacterial mobility.[67]

Because of these complex interactions between the nervous system, immune system, and gut microbe, the importance of behavioral and environmental factors that impact bacterial characteristics in the gut may be greater than previously realized for autoimmune conditions in general, including systemic arthritis. This is further evidence of the interconnection between systems and the impact of a single imbalance on whole body function. The gut-brain may be yet one more mechanism to explain patterns that have long been observable between behaviors such as diet or stress management and an arthritis symptom severity. Further research is needed to determine specifically which bacterial strains may be most implicated in various forms of arthritis, and therefore what interventions via diet or supplementation might be most effective at addressing gut dysbiosis and gut-brain dysfunction. However, it does seem prudent to care for the gut through proper nutrition: limiting inflammatory foods and increasing foods (or perhaps supplements) that support the growth of healthy gut flora. Anyone considering dietary change or supplementation should discuss an individualized approach with a trusted physician or other healthcare professional.

The Role of Yoga Therapy in Healthcare

While some health professionals suggest the avoidance of yoga based on their own assumptions or misinformation, there are genuine cases of concerns about the safety of particular movements for individual patients. It is the responsibility of yoga professionals and practitioners to help inform the medical community about the role of therapeutic yoga and how it differs from standard yoga classes for well populations. To further credit the profession, yoga teachers/therapists should be sensitive to HIPAA privacy laws and follow standard procedures of other healthcare professionals, such as providing progress notes and/or seeking guidance/clarification when appropriate. In addition, be sure to speak with the appropriate medical professional about any specific concerns and how they can be address through the modification of practice or an individual plan of care. Individuals with arthritis can engage their doctor in a conversation about yoga to get a better understanding of what should be avoided or adapted. Yoga professionals can reach out to medical providers for improved communication and collaborative care.

While yoga is currently available in communities throughout the modern Western world, many styles of yoga are rigorous and may be inappropriate for those who require individualized modifications. For example, people with arthritis may have difficulty with bearing weight on or moving affected joints in some directions and may require adaptations of even some basic poses. Yoga for Arthritis instructors are specifically trained to meet the needs and limitations of persons with arthritis. Working with students who have joint disease requires a rudimentary understanding of the disease physiology, as well as more advanced training in joint anatomy than a standard teacher training program offers. Some instructors may have arthritis themselves, experience working with students who have arthritis or additional healthcare training that informs their teaching. Yoga for Arthritis offers continuing education for yoga teachers to support them and people with arthritis in developing healthy, effective practice. You can find a Yoga for Arthritis teacher in your area at www.arthritis.yoga.

Another group with adequate training to meet the needs of people with arthritis may be yoga therapists. Internationally certified yoga therapists require additional in-depth training of at least 1000 hours, compared to the 200 hours needed to become a yoga teacher.[68] The emerging field of yoga therapy emphasizes the individual needs and limitations of each individual and specializes in tailoring yoga practice to address the unique circumstances of each student/client. This may occur in an individual session or in a class for persons who share a common diagnosis, such as arthritis. A yoga therapist may be an ideal place to start, followed by a more general yoga class that moves slowly enough to accommodate individual variations.

Social support and understanding are important for anyone, but especially those with chronic disease; active listening and mindful compassion are important components of healthy support. People with arthritis may be so accustomed to having physical difficulty with tasks that they may be reluctant or fearful about failing at yoga. Because of this, it is important for yoga therapists to stress that there is no "right" way to do a pose. There are many ways that a pose can be beneficial, and you may actually be surprised at how much more is possible by the end of just eight weeks of practice. Some small accomplishments and milestones may help to build self-efficacy and a belief in the ability to achieve and fulfill certain activities or tasks. Yoga professionals should be sure to respect and honor each person's boundaries; if they are not ready to try something, there is a reminder that they can always try it next time, or whenever they feel ready. This accepting approach helps foster a sense of support and understanding and is in accordance with the ethical guidelines of yoga.

Yoga's Ethical Approach to Postures

Each of the ten ethical principles of yoga (*yamas* and *niyamas*) discussed in the previous chapter can be applied to yoga postures just as readily as they can be applied to everyday living. The guiding ethic, non-harm, applies to how the body feels in the postures in addition to the thoughts one thinks during them. Be truthful (*satya*) about the limits of the body and do not steal (*asteya*) wellbeing by being self-critical or pushing too hard. Do not grasp (*aparigraha*) for abilities that are not present in that moment. By accepting things as they are, energy is conserved and directed towards healing (*brahmacharya*), rather than wasted on striving for something that is not there and potentially creating harm. Remember that the purpose of practice is to support health on all levels (*sauca*). Be content with whatever shows up during practice (*samtosha*); balance it with disciplined effort (*tapas*) to keep yoga practice a routine. Study the philosophical aspects of yoga or some other inspirational approach and observe how the teachings relate to your body, energy, emotions, mind, and even spiritual life (*svadhyaya*). Surrender each practice, the events of each day and even the arthritis and its symptoms to a greater reality (*ishvara pranidhana*), knowing that one's human perspective is biased and limited. When you or your clients are aware of these guiding ethics, the entire practice of yoga gains depth, richness, and safety.

Non-Harm (Ahimsa) in Yoga Practice

First, it is a foundational principle of yoga to do no harm (*ahimsa*). While people living with arthritis are often experiencing pain, yoga should not increase or exacerbate that pain. As such, it is important to start by learning to pay attention to physical experience and notice when a practice is increasing arthritis pain. Additionally, it is ideal to start by working with a professional. This might be a yoga therapist or an experienced yoga teacher who works with clinical populations. Such a professional can provide important feedback about safe alignment, make recommendations for adapting the practice and ensure that a student is oriented to the underlying philosophy that will optimize benefit and minimize harms. As with any new activity, it is important to speak with any medical doctors providing ongoing care to get suggestions about movements or positions to avoid. A yoga therapist might even want to speak directly with a client's physical therapist, or receive a list of contraindicated positions from a medical specialist. Ultimately, of course, the world's leading expert of a particular body is the person living within it. Above all else, trust that experience and honor its wisdom.

One might suggest that if a yogi suffers harm from yoga practice, it wasn't really yoga. In other words, when you are engaged in a practice of non-harming, harms should be avoided. However, we know that sometimes people do experience harms during yoga practice. Research suggests that yoga interventions are as safe as educational programs or usual care but the yoga programs in research studies are thoughtfully developed, expertly delivered, and highly supervised. Risks may differ in community-based programs.

In addition to the precautions recommended to avoid physical harm during yoga practice, it is important to consider that yoga is a whole-person experience. Just as many aspects of the self may experience benefits from practice, they must also be protected from harm. Yoga is a practice that invites participants to get quiet, go within, and pay attention to what comes up. Sometimes the observations will be physical (I feel my quadriceps engaged) and sometimes it will be mental (I am worried about becoming disabled) or spiritual (why me?). Just as with physical sensation, observe the experience with playful curiosity (isn't that interesting?!), but also assure safety for yourself and others. Remember that arthritis is associated with other medical conditions and risk factors, in both physical and mental health. If someone with arthritis (or anyone for that matter) feels unsafe physically, mentally, emotionally, or otherwise, it is not yoga. If you are uncomfortable with a practice or experience, decide whether it is just a curious sensation that you can ride through and observe, or whether it is making you feel unsafe. Just as you are the world's leading expert of your own body, you are also the only one who can decide if your mental/emotional state is being challenged safely or unsafely. You have the right to say no to any potential harm. By making non-harm the guiding principle of yoga practice, you are ensuring it is truly a yogic experience.

Joint Modifications and Adaptations

There are many common guidelines for keeping joints safe during an *asana* practice. The best gauge is your body's own messages. Someone who is uncertain about how far to go into a posture can err on the side of caution, gradually deepening poses over time and with a mindful approach. If you have arthritis in any of the following joints, here are things to consider. For a full exposition of modifications, please visit the Appendix.

Spine

It is most important for the spine to maintain its length and natural curvatures. In seated postures, this is easiest if a person sits on a block or cushion on the points of the sitz bones. Be sure that in both flexion and extension that the spine is not kinking in a particular spot; rather, the curve is even along the spine's length. You may imagine forming the back over a ball or a geometric protractor instead of creating a "break" or angular bend at a specific location in the back. A soft bend in the knees further reduces the demand upon the back. Do not use the arms to force a twist in the back or to press into a backbend; allow the strength and movement to come from the torso and use the hands and arms only for support.

Neck

Be sure not to hyperextend or flex the neck. Do not drop the head backward. Be sure that there is muscular control when tilting the head back. You may even support the head with the hands and gaze slightly upward (where ceiling and wall meet) instead of looking directly up.

Shoulders

In some cases, it may be prudent to keep the arms lower than shoulder height. Even if it is comfortable to raise the arms overhead, be sure to keep the shoulders mobile, not compressed or tense, as the arms come up. The arms may be in a wide "V" overhead or with elbows bent. In time, the biceps might come closer to the ears while keeping the shoulder blades relaxed down the back.

Elbows

As with all joints, be sure not to lock the elbows, which is a hyperextension of the joint and an unstable position. Think of keeping a slight bend and notice the strength in the muscles through the arms. Be mindful of elbows, especially with poses that require weight-bearing through the arms. Consider using a wall or chair for support instead of doing the pose on the floor at first.

Wrists

Many people with arthritis have great sensitivity in the wrists. There are numerous adaptations to keep this joint safe and comfortable. Instead of flattening the palms on the floor, which can be an extreme angle for the wrist, try coming onto fists or forearms placed on blocks/chair. Alternatively, a wedge or folded towel can be placed beneath the palms to make the bend more accessible.

Hands

Similar to the issues with the wrists, the hands may be too sensitive to perform weight-bearing postures. Options listed above for the wrists may also help the hands. One may place the forearms on a block and hang the hands over the edge. Experiment with different ways of holding the hands. Some people may prefer to interlace fingers, or press palms, while others would rather hold a wrist in the hand and then change sides. *Mudra* can be challenging for the hands, so be mindful of that and adapt as needed. Be sure to mobilize the hands to avoid stiffness, without overusing them.

Hips

The hips are involved in many yoga postures. It is best to limit the amount of pressure on the hips while they are stretching, which might mean changing the orientation of the posture for example from seated, with legs on the mat, to reclined, with legs in the air. Reducing flexion and external rotation of the hips can create more ease, and sitting in a chair instead of on the floor may be preferable.

Knees

Be mindful not to hyperextend or twist the knee. Keep knees aligned with ankles or hips; if knees move out in front of the toes, adjust the stance so that the feet are placed beneath the knees. Similar to the elbows, it is best to have a slight bend in the knee and perceive the leg muscles supporting the pose. In postures where the knee is bearing weight, be sure to have a good amount of cushion beneath the joint, such as folded blankets. It is also an option to forego knee-down postures and do them seated or standing against a wall instead.

Ankles

The wedging methods used for the wrists can also benefit the ankles. Placing a wedge or folded blanket beneath the heels helps lessen the demand at this lower joint and offers greater support. Some poses require the ankles to be at angles not used in daily life. It is fine to choose a different orientation for the ankle in such cases.

Feet

Yoga is traditionally performed barefoot. While some people might experience this as freeing, others require the support of athletic footwear. It can be beneficial to practice at least a little bit in bare feet in order to increase proprioception and possibly limit the risk of falls as the feet become more sensitive to the connection to the ground. Whether in shoes or not, attempt to spread the weight throughout the foot and experiment with lifting the arches and pressing front, side and back to experiment with different ways of standing.

There are as many options for modifying postures as there are people performing them. Let this brief list be a starting point for you as you come to understand the key aspects of joint safety in yoga for arthritis. Explore the Appendix for more details.

Beyond Posture Modifications

The poses described in this book are usually modified from the "classical" form. But the modifications are not the point. Instead, I like to think that we are using modifications so that the postures are accessible, and then the real yoga takes place.

In order to modify, one may use props, shortened range of movement or other adaptations like those listed above to make adjustments as you/your clients learn self-care through yoga. Arthritis symptoms vary, which means it is important to experiment with a range of modifications in postures. From there, a yoga therapist or qualified yoga teacher can find versions of each *asana* that remain true to the spirit of the pose.

It is important to identify the "essence" of each yoga pose. Seeking your own underlying intention or becoming aware of the specific attitude (*bhavana*) or archetype of the *asana* is beneficial. Remember, a yoga pose is a physical position that creates a certain state of mind. You might ask, "Why am I including this pose in the practice?" Each pose can have multiple intentions. It might be something physical about the pose, like lengthening the hamstrings or strengthening the adductors. It might be energetic, like creating a sense of calm, or mental, like harnessing inner conviction. Whatever the purpose of the pose in that moment, there is a way to make that accessible to absolutely anyone. The method might be a simple and minor adjustment, like placing a wedge under the palms to reduce wrist flexion, or it might mean turning a standing pose into something lying on the floor. There is no single correct answer and each situation offers multiple options. Try not to get hung up on the shape of the pose. Two versions of a pose might look completely different but achieve the same intention, while two similar-looking poses might be very different in intention, energy, or even physical effects. Anyone with a body and mind can practice yoga, regardless of limitations or abilities, and every pose has some version that can be accessible to the individual student.

When we think about bringing the tools of yoga to the arthritis community, yoga professionals should look beyond the modification of *asana* as a goal. The goal instead is to make the *asanas* possible, so the totality of yoga can come through, safely and effectively. Additionally, share the wisdom and experience of yoga's more subtle aspects to improve lives in many dimensions of experience.

Noticing Sensations and Responding to Pain

Throughout this book, I remind you to listen to your body, or to encourage your patients/clients to do the same. People may not always want to pay attention to the body's signals. When one lives with chronic pain, it seems necessary to disregard it in order to function in everyday life. However, in order to practice non-harm, one must remain aware. Any movements that increase pain should be avoided or highly limited.

Sometimes it can be challenging to interpret the signals from the body. I discuss pain perception more in Chapters 6 and 7. Note that there is a difference between pain and sensation. If you experience chronic pain, you may have learned to ignore a certain level or dismiss it as normal. Please be sure to err on the side of caution when you begin yoga. Avoid pain as much as possible.

When attempting a new activity, such as yoga, it is natural to experience sensation and discomfort. Strengthening muscles may send a signal of burning. Stretching muscles may tingle or pull. These signals are not the same as arthritic joint pain. Encourage clients to ask, "Where am I feeling this? Is it in my joints, the tendons at the end of the muscle or in the 'belly' of the muscle, where I have the greatest capacity to stretch and strengthen?"

Also notice the quality of the sensation. Is it a dull ache or a sharp, shooting pain? Where the former may be a natural aspect of increasing physical fitness, the latter is likely a warning sign that the movement or position should be stopped or altered immediately. Pain will make you grimace or reach for the hurt part of the body. It may even show up as a numbing. Remember that there are a variety of options for any given pose. None of these options is better than another, beyond what is best for an individual student.

As people practice yoga, the skill of mindfulness develops. In time, it becomes easier to discern the difference between pain and sensation. Messages from the body seem clearer and the prudent options for response are also more familiar. The story around the pain becomes less elaborate as people simply adapt and move on, without creating a mental stress. For example, the skill of noticing how the quadriceps feel in Chair Pose is the same whether a person is fatigued, achy, strong, or inflamed on any given day. There is no need to project into the past or fear the future based on the messages from the quads; simply notice and adapt as required. Yoga builds the ability to observe with non-judgment and act with discernment.

Summary

Obesity, disability, and sedentary lifestyle are all physical issues impacting people with arthritis. Yoga is an adaptable, accessible form of mental and physical activity that supports whole-person wellness. The physical components of yoga can be approached safely by anyone, under the proper guidance of a trained yoga professional. Yoga is not static, and the practice can be adapted to changes in health and joint activity. With proper professional guidance, it is possible for persons with arthritis to develop a life-long yoga practice that is safe, convenient, and adaptable to disease-related changes in physical function. As one becomes established in yoga, the more subtle benefits become evident.

Chapter 5

THE ENERGY LAYER (*PRANAMAYA KOSHA*)

The following chapter explores PMK, or the energetic sheath of yoga's PMK model. This is the layer of being that relates to the breath and the movement of subtle energy, similar to the meridian system in acupuncture and Traditional Chinese Medicine. In this chapter, I discuss healthy breath and basic energy anatomy and give you the opportunity to experience aspects of your own PMK.

The Healing Power of Breath

The abdominal diaphragm is a dome-shaped organ that separates the upper and lower organs within the torso. It is one of multiple diaphragms in the body but is generally referred to as "the diaphragm." Above the diaphragm are the heart and lungs, while below it are the digestive organs. When we inhale and the chest fills with air, the lungs and ribcage expand. For a fuller, deeper breath than the chest cavity alone can allow, the diaphragm descends and moves the digestive organs out of the way to create more space for the inhalation. When we exhale, the lungs empty and the diaphragm moves upward. This is why the belly expands when we inhale—the diaphragm has pushed the contents of the lower abdomen downward, which then temporarily expand outward. As we exhale, there is more space in the lower abdomen and the belly moves back inward.

You can observe this by placing a hand on your belly. Check to see whether it expands outward when you breathe in. Some call this "diaphragmatic breathing" because the diaphragm is moving up and down with each breath. Some people have a breath pattern that is shallow and only expanding the chest cavity, while others have a "reverse-breathing" pattern, where the abdomen rises on the exhale and contracts on the inhale. These other ways of breathing can exacerbate stress, anxiety, and depression and do not allow for the full exchange of oxygen and waste products from the bloodstream that full breathing fosters. While some people are concerned that the belly protruded with each inhale, this is actually an abdominal workout! Think of each in and out breath as an exercise for the abdominal muscles that increase in tone with each full breath.

But there is another important way that breathing and health are linked. The diaphragm is enervated by a two-nerve system called the vagus nerve. The vagus nerve is the longest nerve in the body and gets its name from its wandering pattern through various body systems. The vagus nerve is involved with regulation of the ANS, which regulates the stress and relaxation response. We know that the stress response has several physiological components, including increased heart rate, dilated pupils, reduced digestion, changed blood flow, and more. The vagus nerve connects with these many different body systems, such as the heart, the eyes, the stomach, among others. As the diaphragm ascends and descends with each breath, it interacts with the vagus nerve and affects ANS function.

As a result, there is a pattern in a healthy heart rate that involves a slight speeding up with each inhale and a slight slowing with each exhale. The SNS is engaged on the inhale and the PNS is engaged in the exhale. This is part of what we call *heart rate variability* (HRV). HRV is the ability of our body to adjust and adapt to changes in our environment. Our heart rate should speed up when we see a bear and slow down when we realize it is headed away from us. HRV is an incredibly accurate marker of overall health and health risk.

Because of this pattern, we can use the breath to affect the nervous system. You may have noticed these effects already by practicing the Balanced Breath in Chapter 2 or the Three-Part Breath in Chapter 3. When we alter our breathing patterns, we impact the nervous system. By spending more time on the exhale, for example, we can engage the relaxation response. The more time we spend exhaling, the more our heart rate has a chance to slow and relax, taking us out of the stress response that is associated with greater pain and less joy. Greater PNS activation can help reduce pain and inflammation, improve sleep, and ease our psychological concerns.

It is also important to consider the impact of various breathing patterns during physical activity. Most people think of aerobic exercise as being limited to activities such as running, cycling, swimming, and the like. In fact, aerobic exercise is any exercise that is fully supported by sufficient oxygenation. Exercise such as weightlifting is considered anaerobic and relies on stored glycogen to support the activity. A byproduct of this process is lactic acid, which can be associated with muscle soreness. Additionally, when glycogen stores are used up, exercisers often "hit a wall" of fatigue.

Any activity moves from being aerobic to anaerobic when it is too strenuous or oxygenation is insufficient. For example, if you were trying to keep up with an Olympic athlete, cycling would become anaerobic. The same is true if you are not getting the full oxygenation that deep breathing during exercise can afford. Full breathing, as described in the three-part breath exercise of Chapter 3, allows for greater oxygen exchange and keeps activity aerobic instead of anaerobic, reducing the likelihood of lactic acid build-up and fatigue from glycogen depletion. Depending on your fitness level, this could happen during activities of various intensity levels. Whether you are taking a brisk walk or practicing yoga, be sure to notice your breath.

Noticing the breath in everyday moments also supports the overall health of the nervous system and can be highly beneficial to people with arthritis. A complete breath—where the respiratory diaphragm is properly mobilized, the intercostal muscles expand to the front, sides, and back, and the chest blooms open—sends an immediate message through the ANS: be calm. This healing energy of peacefulness, throughout the body's systems as well as the mind and emotions, is a foundation for easing the symptoms of arthritis.

The concept of PMK teaches that the layer within the physical self is the animating force: breath and the lifeforce energy carried on the breath. All living things breathe. We can see the body physically breathing through the movement of its organs and muscles, but the breath's energy (*prana*) is unseen.

Does Subtle Energy Exist?

Western models of health and healing lack constructs for energy centers (*chakras*) and channels (*nadis*) which carry the life force. Perhaps for that reason, Western science does not have tools for measuring the body's energetic field. In other words, *prana*, or "life force" doesn't show up on an MRI. Of course, not everything that is real is visible to the human eye. Depression is a good example. We cannot see mood, but we know it exists and we have developed methods for measuring it because that is important for diagnosis and treatment. We also know that changes in mood have a measurable impact on biological systems. We can see, for example, that depression is associated with specific changes in brain activity that *can* be seen on MRI. Mood also impacts other body systems and most certainly it impacts behavior.

While it may feel like a stretch to conceive of invisible energy channels in the body, the map of these centers and channels originated thousands of years ago in yoga. They are very similar to the meridians and points used in acupuncture and Chinese Medicine. Acupuncture stimulates these points to impact the flow of energy through the body. In yoga, this energy is called *prana*; in Chinese Medicine it is called *Qi* or *Chi*. Yoga does not use needles to stimulate the flow of *prana*; rather, breath and movement techniques are practiced for shifting energy, similar to the use of *Tai Chi* and *Qi gong* in Chinese culture.

Of these modalities, acupuncture has been the most studied most via Western scientific methodology. Unfortunately, Western research methods were designed to test the effects of a drug on health outcomes and are not well suited to measure a treatment such as acupuncture. The use of a double-blind, placebo-controlled trial, which is the gold standard in modern medicine, requires that both the doctor and the patient are not aware of whether they are receiving the drug. That works fine when comparing a drug to a sugar pill, but it isn't possible for an acupuncturist or her patient to be unaware that the treatment is happening. Strategies to develop a "sham acupuncture" for comparison have been imperfect at best.[69] Some of the problem is that the *context* of the treatment and the experience the patient is having outside of just the needle is an important part of acupuncture care. For example, the acupuncturists' intention, which cannot be easily measured, is thought to impact treatment.

Despite all of these challenges, acupuncture research has grown in sophistication in recent years and has shown consistent effects for some outcomes, especially for pain.[70] The greatest resistance to acupuncture in the medical community for a long time was the lack of understanding about how it worked. It is now becoming more common for medical doctors to say, "I don't know how it works, but it seems to work." In fact, many Western medical doctors are incorporating acupuncture techniques into medical practice. The effectiveness of acupuncture, as evidenced by many years of accumulating research evidence, is best explained by a system of energy channels and centers, even if we can't see them. Some scientists are working on ways to measure the energy in those points and channels through magnetic field measurement, although the evidence has not been overwhelming or conclusive yet.

Is it possible that acupuncture works even in the absence of the energy channels and points that form its basis? Sure. But despite many bright minds working on the subject, we have yet to find a clear alternative hypothesis for its mechanisms. Consider taking a leap of faith that thousands of years of work across multiple cultures (Tibetan Medicine uses energy channels also) and decades of modern science are in alignment. Once you start to pay attention, you will probably find that you can notice changes in your own energy field. You might even be able to notice an opening or restriction in some energy centers that can't be explained by muscular action. Indeed, you might begin to sense that your "self" exists beyond the limits of your physical body, and that you feel an energy field outside of your own skin.

SENSE YOUR ENERGY *KOSHA*

The following exercise gives you the opportunity to explore how you or anyone else might interact with the energy layer. Try it yourself and/or share it with others. Have fun with this and use your imagination. Give your mind some space to be calm and uplifted. (You may perform the Heart Relaxation in this chapter for a relaxing practice before beginning.)

1. Stand in a stable position, with feet planted at least shoulder-width apart, feeling grounded and rested. Without changing it, notice the depth, rhythm, pace, and quality of your breath. How smooth is it? If your breathing changes of its own volition, allow it. All you have to do is notice the breath.

2. Clap your hands together a few times and observe the sensation that follows. It may feel warm, tingly, numb, strong… Acknowledge any images, memories or emotions that come to mind. Notice your breath.

3. Rub your hands together to create heat then pull your palms apart slowly. Sense the continuing connection between your hands, even though they are no longer physically touching. What messages are your nerves sending and receiving? Do you perceive warmth, tingling, or a sense of repulsion or attraction? If each palm were a magnet, would they be pulling toward or pushing away from one another?

4. Explore the space between the palms with each of your five senses. You may "see" a color swirling there or "feel" a texture. If you lose that sense of connection between the palms, repeat Steps 2 and 3 then tap into each of your five senses as you hold your attention on the space between your palms or fingertips.

5. Repeats Steps 2 and 3 again. This time, select a joint that sometimes "speaks" to you and place your palm(s) on/around it. Notice the sense of physical or energetic connection there. You may imagine a healing color or feeling flowing into that joint, cooling, lubricating, and soothing it. Repeat this step for as many areas as you wish.

This exercise gave you the chance to experiment with your subtle perceptions and work with your energy layer. Now that you have a way of exploring PMK, you may use it to investigate the subtleties of what may be happening within your body when you feel healthy and during flares. This understated method of perception may make you more sensitive to noticing flares, fatigue, pain, and other symptoms sooner as you remain attuned to your subtle senses.

RELAXATION: HEART RELAXATION

Yoga professionals can read this to a client or a class. Others may want to record this and play it for themselves, or ask someone to read it to you while you relax. As mentioned previously, it is normal for emotions to surface when we slow down and focus inwards. These are useful messages and you do not have to react to them in relaxation. It is okay to just notice the effect on your breath, body, and sense of relaxation:

1. Bring yourself into a comfortable lying position. You may want to place some support or cushioning under your knees, the back of your neck or anywhere that would provide more comfort to the joints. If you feel the desire to make an adjustment to the body during this relaxation, feel free to do so. The goal is to be more relaxed, and that means honoring your inner teacher about what adjustments might be helpful. Try to do this in a quiet place where you can be without distraction for a few minutes.

2. Begin by noticing all the parts of your body that are supported by the surface beneath you. Allow your body to become heavy and to melt into that support. Consider all of the support that is available to you in life—friends, family, colleagues, neighbors… Rest in the knowing that support is available to you, even if you don't always allow yourself to be supported. Let this moment be an opportunity to let go, without any obligations or demands. Allow yourself to just be, without doing—a necessity in the cycle of energy that moves between exertion and recuperation. The more you do, the more you must allow yourself the opportunity to rest, reflect, recover, and renew. This relaxation is a practice of renewal.

3. Notice any parts of the body that are holding tension or muscle engagement. Remind those body parts that you are safe and it is okay to let go of their holding patterns. Now is a time to rest and release. Begin at the toes and slowly relax every part of the body—the feet and ankles, the leg and pelvis, the belly and chest. Relax the hands, the arms, the neck, and head. Let the whole body be relaxed.

4. Now become aware of your breath. Notice the rhythm of your breath as it rises and falls. How would you describe your breath right now? Is it fast or slow? Shallow or deep? Faint or strong? What parts of your body expand as you breathe? Can you feel your chest rise and fall? Does your ribcage expand? Is your belly moving with each inhale and exhale? Whatever the nature of your breath in this moment, thank your breath for sustaining you—for continuing unceasingly, even when you sleep. Whatever breathing challenges you may experience or assistance you may need, your breath is your life force and it has never given up on its responsibility to keep you alive. It is the breath that moves energy through the body, that oxygenates all of your cells, bringing nourishment and removing toxicity. Each breath is a process that cleanses the body.

5. There is also an energy to your nervous system. It decides whether you are alert or relaxed. Allow your breath to tell your body that it can relax. A deep breath lets your body know that it is safe. A slow exhale turns on the body's inner relaxation process. Begin to deepen your breath gradually, without forcing. Let the breath grow so that you feel the torso expand in all directions with each inhale and with each slow, easy exhale, you sink deeper into relaxation. Imagine that the breath is not contained to your torso, but that your whole body is breathing in rhythm. Instead of controlling the breath, allow yourself to be breathed. Imagine that you are carried away on a blanket of easeful, peaceful breath.

6. Become aware now of your heart—the home of unconditional love, joy, and serenity. Whatever feelings may have arisen in your heart in the past, you are safe in this relaxation and can allow your heart to soften and expand. Your heart is the source of compassion and connection within yourself and with all living things you encounter. Your heart is the knower of truths that the mind cannot explain or understand. Perhaps you connect with your heart often and listen to its wisdom. Perhaps your heart is sometimes a source of sadness and is in need of healing. Allow the breath to fill your heart with healing and renewal, as it does for all the cells of the body. Feel the heart strengthen as it is nourished by the fullness of your breath.

7. In the womb, the heart and hands emerge from the same embryonic tissue. There is an integral connection between the love of the heart and the action of the hands. Allow your actions in the world to be informed by the love and compassion in your heart. Feel the kindness of the heart spreading out to the hands and nourishing them. Allow the warmth of the heart to expand through the whole body, filling you with love and light. Imagine that your body is enveloped in a heart-centered love that expands beyond your physical form and into the space around you. Let yourself be nourished by this love and rest in the comfort of your heart's wisdom.

8. Spend a few moments just enjoying this experience. Let yourself relax in this space of loving kindness, of gentle relaxation, of nourishing breath. (Allow a minute or so of silence here.)

9. Begin allowing your breath to deepen once again, bringing energy and vitality to all parts of the body. Even with your eyes still closed, become

aware of your body and the space around you. Move any parts of your body that are ready to move, slowly wiggling or rocking side to side. Perhaps take a big stretch in any direction and roll onto one side for a few more breaths. Gently bring yourself up to sitting and take a moment to notice the effects of this relaxation. Notice the ease in the body, fullness in the breath, openness in the heart, clarity in the mind.

Know that this is available to you anytime and return to it as often as you like. Thank yourself for taking this time for self-care, and for bringing the benefits of this relaxation into the rest of your day. Namaste.

Brahmacharya: Right Use of Energy

A key practice in Classical yoga is the conservation or right use of energy (*brahmacharya*). This approach is part of the *yamas,* or ethical restraints. Traditionally, the practitioner directs all energies toward the Divine, often including the practice of celibacy, but that concept can also be interpreted much more broadly in how we use our energy optimally. *Brahmacharya* means not wasting energy on worry, digesting junk foods, overextending oneself, and other common habits that leave us feeling fatigued or unhealthy. Furthermore, we help conserve our vital energy through proper activity, nutrition, reading uplifting materials, music, meaningful company, and other habits and routines that connect us to a sense of peace and purpose. It can be thought of as "right" use of energy, including a focus on thoughts, words, and actions that best serve our health and priorities. This concept is particularly important when the challenges of managing arthritis can require so much energy, and the symptom of fatigue can mean less energy available for daily life.

REFLECTION: REFLECTION ON ENERGY

The following reflection questions help to evaluate one's practice of conserving or directing energy. You or your clients can answer these questions in a journal and observe related habits over the next couple of weeks. These questions may be revisited a few times per year and they should get careful attention at the beginning of a flare. Because *brahmacharya* deals with subtle energies, the effects of our lifestyle choices show up in quiet ways such as more relaxed responses or a deeper sense of faith or wellbeing. One might not notice the understated effects without actively seeking them.

REFLECTION QUESTION #1: NUTRITION

How do you cook? Is it daily? In batches? Do you enjoy the process or is it a major life stressor? Is someone else preparing the food? Is food preparation in your home a source of conflict? Is meal time enjoyable? Is it rushed? Distracted? How could food preparation and meal time be more nourishing and less depleting?

What are your typical food selections? Is there a type of food or flavor that draws your attention? Are most of your food choices nourishing or depleting? How do you feel after you eat? Have you noticed any foods that make you feel better or others that make you feel worse afterward? What is one small change you would like to make in your daily dietary habits?

Now, acknowledge the things you are doing that do not serve your health related to your dietary choices. Free yourself from judgment—this is not about sorting "good" and "bad" choices. Simply acknowledge the habits and choices that may be wasting your precious energy.

REFLECTION QUESTION #2: REST

Everyone has a different pattern of exertion and recuperation. The easiest example of this is our sleep-wake patterns. After being awake (exerting) for hours, the body needs to sleep (recuperate). But there are many other ways that we exert and recuperate over the short and long term.

First, are you getting enough sleep? Is it good quality sleep? Are your room, bed, and home conducive to quality sleep? Is there anything you could do to optimize your sleep time and environment?

In your daily life, do you take moments to recuperate? Examples might be making a cup of tea, stepping outdoors, getting up from your desk, taking a few deep breaths, even a short nap. Do you go long periods without a break? If so, what effect does that have on your energy? Do you get an opportunity for some "down time" at the beginning or end of your day? Time with loved ones or in solitude without demands? What does that look like? What effect does it have on your energy?

Think about the pattern of your typical week. Do you observe a day of rest, either secular or religious? Do you have time away from technology and/or work? Is there special time for family or friends built into your week? If so, what effect does that have on your energy? Is there any time in your week for quiet reflection?

What about your year? Do you take vacations? "Staycations"? Are there times of the year that are particularly full or stressful? If so, can that be changed? Otherwise, do you have an opportunity to recover from your most challenging times of year? How might this be built in to your calendar somehow?

REFLECTION QUESTION #3: RELATIONSHIPS

Who in your life gets most of your time and energy? Who makes you laugh? Who encourages you? Who can you vent to? Are there people in your life who deplete your energy? If so, what could you do to minimize the impact? Are there some relationships that aren't serving you and that you could let go of? Are there a few people closest to you who bring you the most joy? Do you have a support network that you can rely on for times when you feel fatigued or overwhelmed? Oftentimes, people with arthritis find themselves pruning relationships to focus on the most meaningful ones, perhaps considering who are the most honest, reliable, and nourishing people in their lives. Are you able to make time for the relationships that fill your tank instead of the ones that deplete you? There is a wonderful quote on this topic in a poem by David Whyte called *Sweet Darkness*. The end of the poem reads:

> Sometimes it takes darkness and the sweet
> confinement of your aloneness
> to learn
>
> anything or anyone
> that does not bring you alive
>
> is too small for you.

You might consider who and what "brings you alive" and how that awareness might affect your future choices.

REFLECTION QUESTION #4: ACTIVITIES

What media do you consume? What do you look forward to? When do you feel most yourself? Are you doing things you don't want to? Are there commitments you made out of a sense of obligation that deplete you? Are there any that you could let go of? What would be the consequences? Do you have criteria for which activities you will agree to take on? Have you allowed those criteria to change over time as needed?

Are there activities in your life that bring you the most joy? That energize you? Are there obligations that you could pass on, delegate, or share with someone else? When you make a commitment, do you feel comfortable retracting it when the circumstances change? Or do you feel obligated no matter the circumstances? Do the people in your life understand your disease and the sometimes unexpected impact it can have on your energy or ability to follow-through with commitments? How could you have those conversations in an honest, authentic, respectful, and meaningful way? Again, David Whyte's lines from *Sweet Darkness* seem pertinent here.

Through a habit of saying yes, or a lack of attention to pruning our lives, we often wind up with too many things on the go at once. We can't let go of all distasteful responsibilities but we can delegate or get help. In the case of housework, for example, it is recommended that children as young as three or four years old begin taking on household responsibilities within their capabilities. Over the course of the next month, evaluate all the demands on your time. Which of these agenda items can you let go or pare down? In some cases, you may need to create a plan to extricate yourself over time.

REFLECTION QUESTION #5: KEY INDICATORS

The next time you feel fatigued, ask yourself if there was a sign you were about to get tired. Before you were smacked with tiredness, were there inklings of fatigue? Did you make choices based on having low energy? You can apply this inquiry to your energetic patterns across a 24-hour period in order to identify your peak productivity and most important resting times.

When do you feel most enlivened? Most productive? When is it challenging to accomplish things? Is it harder to move at certain times of day? More importantly, this reflection question can help you learn the signs that you are headed for an arthritis flare. At first, you may notice that right before a flare you stop cooking for yourself or doing dishes. Later, you may notice that you had stopped flossing your teeth a few days before that. The next time, you might observe that forgoing the weekly wash of bed sheets preceded the decline in oral hygiene. All of these are signs that you can use to help make choices with greater awareness and conserve your energy.

REFLECTION QUESTION #6: OPTIONS

What is the first thing you do when you notice an uptick in your symptoms? Do you call your doctor? Cancel your plans? Ignore it? Do you take more medicine? Use ice or heat? Get extra sleep? What are the consequences of those choices? What feelings arise? Denial? Frustration? Acceptance? Fear? Do you tell anyone or keep it to yourself? Are there ways you could respond to your symptoms that would be more optimal for recovery and wellness? Is there anything you could change in your life right now that might help to prevent or reduce major fluctuations in your symptoms?

There is a poem by Mary Oliver entitled "The Summer Day" that ends with the two lines, "Tell me, what is it you plan to do/with your one wild and precious life?"[71] I often think of these lines when discussing the concept of *bramacharya* with clients. If energy, resources or time is limited, the importance of wise use comes to the fore. There are even watches on the market that countdown to the estimated end of life in order to remind us that every moment counts. While no one would wish for fatigue, it can foster a kind of refocusing on what truly matters in life, and even sometimes an appreciation for having made those deliberate choices.

There are always more clues about how to improve health than we initially realize. There are a multitude of ways you can take greater control of your schedule, emotions, and wellbeing to conserve and channel your energy, even if it seems like your life has many constraints. By completing these reflection questions, you are on the path of understanding more about how you are directing your energy, as well as opportunities to conserve it. Attention to cultivating healthy energy is a key component of yoga practice.

Practices to Boost Energy

Yoga offers many tools to balance and enhance healthy energy. The following practices are recommended to energize you or those you work with. Please note that fatigue may be a cue to rest, rather than resist and attempt to increase energy. Through mindfulness, the distinction will become clear. There is a difference between practices to lift one out of fatigue and practices that are modified because one *is* fatigued. This section addresses the former. I cover the latter in the following chapter.

As you make yoga practices a part of everyday life, it is important to have a home sanctuary that can be a place of respite and recovery. It may be a dedicated practice room, a bedroom, or just a quiet, pleasant corner of your home. It might even be a walk-in closet or the floor of the laundry room. You just need enough space to lie down and stretch out without distraction. You may customize this practice space with sacred objects, art, black-out shades, soothing music, and calming scents. It is important that you are able to regulate the temperature, so have blankets and a fan nearby. Be selective about your color choices, if possible, and keep clutter to a minimum. If you live with others, you may create a signal or sign that you are taking time for self-care so that they know not to disturb you during practice.

The typical safety guidelines apply to the following practices. Trust yourself and listen to your body, discerning between sensation and pain. Do not push through your body's warning signs. Remember that these practices are meant to be energizing. If they have the opposite effect and make you feel more fatigued, that may be a sign that it is important to rest and perform the practices in the following chapter instead. Enjoy the opportunity to connect to your body, energy, and mind as you dedicate time to your wellbeing.

BREATHING: BREATH OF FIRE (*KAPALABHATI PRANAYAMA*)

The following breathing practice, *kapalabhati*, is a terrific "fatigue-buster." It is not appropriate during flares, as it is a heating practice, but it is excellent when one needs an energy boost. I know people who like to use it instead of a morning cup of coffee, or in the afternoon when energy levels often wane. Some people even head to the bathroom at work or school for a few rejuvenating rounds of this breath before heading back to the task at hand. Rest anytime you feel fatigued or dizzy, simply breathing normally. Ironically, it is common for some people to feel fatigued by this practice, which is a clear sign that rest is needed. Trust your body's need for rest and do not force *kapalabhati* in hopes that it will bring you energy when you actually need a break. Otherwise, enjoy the practice as a way of inciting vitality.

Begin with a slow, full inhale. Notice as you flex the abdominals firmly inward the diaphragm presses up, which in turn forces the air from the lungs. Use this abdominal action to expel the air. You may attempt this for ten contractions or continue until the lungs feel empty. When you relax, the lungs will naturally fill again. Repeat this slow inhale, bursting exhales a few times to become comfortable with the vigorous expulsion of air. I recommend you attempt this practice for ten breaths to begin with. In time, you may increase to a full *kapalabhati* breath pattern and maintain it for two or three minutes. If this is difficult to conceptualize, try doing an online search for videos of this breath. You will probably find that the example of someone else doing it is clearer than the explanation. If you are not used to intentionally controlling your breath, it may seem odd. Approach it playfully as an experiment to see what happens and how it makes you feel.

Now that you have experimented with an energizing breath, you have a pick-me-up tool. Practice *kapalabhati* to energize yourself through breath. The following yoga pose practice can invigorate you by moving the body.

POSTURE: SUN SALUTATION *VINYASA* SUPPORTED BY A CHAIR

A *vinyasa* practice is series of yoga postures linked together so that they create a fluid movement sequence. The most popular *vinyasa* is the Sun Salutation (*Surya Namaskara*). Variations of this sequence are found in most contemporary styles of yoga. Images of options for Sun Salutation can be found in the Appendix. The following practice is modified using a chair to support the various positions. To practice Sun Salutation while seated in a chair, please see the Chapter 11. This flowing sequence of poses helps create energy by taking the body through a series of complementary yet gentle movements. When energy is low, it feels good to engage with movement at an empowering level. You may be more aware of your breath as you move through this sequence because it may become labored with the physical effort. This is a terrific opportunity to notice the choices you are making around breath. In what ways can you alter your breathing in order to give you more energy? This query can help you exert yourself in a safe way because the breath is a reliable gauge for an appropriate level of exertion. It's okay if you feel a little winded—that means your heart and lungs are getting stronger— but you must be able to control the breath by slowing it down or modifying it according to your own choice:

1. Place a sturdy chair at the front of your mat and stand in front of it. If the seat of the chair is facing you, the postures will be deeper. If you use the back of the chair for support, instead, then the poses will not be as deep. Spread your weight across the soles of the feet, create length in the spine and keep the chin parallel to the floor. Deepen your breath and place your palms together at the center of your chest or palms on your chest.

2. Inhale and raise the arms to a comfortable height, opening the chest and heart gently.

3. Exhale and fold over the chair. Bring hands to the back or seat of the chair. Knees are soft, not locked, and weight is toward the balls of the feet while the heels remain down.

4. Inhale and step the left foot back as far as is comfortable, coming into a lunge. Be sure that the shoulders are over the hips and knee over the ankle (not past it) as you use the chair for support. Feel the stretch through the back, left leg.

5. Exhale and step the front foot back to a version of Downward-Facing Dog. The hips reach back away from the arms. It is okay to keep the knees soft as you lengthen and feel yourself becoming strong.

6. Inhale. Step both feet forward and bring the hips toward the chair as you arch the back and open through the front of the body. The more forward you step, the more gentle the Cobra posture. From here, repeat each posture in reverse sequence.

7. Transition through an exhale back into Downward-Facing Dog, as in Step 5.

8. Like the pose in Step 4, inhale and step the left foot forward to lunge on the other side, looking forward.

9. The back, right, foot steps forward to fold over the chair on an exhale, similar to Step 3.

10. Inhale as arms raise upward and arch gently back just from the shoulder blades up.

11. Exhale to center. Notice any changes in physical sensation, breath, emotions, and thoughts. Tune in to your sense of energy. Where is there tingling or a feeling of spaciousness? Are there differences in temperature?

12. Repeat the sequence again, this time leading with the right foot. You may repeat the sun salutation sequence several times or use it as a warm-up before moving on to other postures.

Use this practice anytime you are looking for a warm-up, a fluid sequence, or an opportunity to energize yourself.

Summary

In this chapter, I discussed the breath/energy layer, *PMK*. The PMK model reminds us to consider and respond to our health needs beyond the obvious physical plane. By attuning to the breath and inner experiences, people with arthritis may be better able to respond to shifts in energy levels. The practices in this chapter help bring balance, whether energizing or relaxing, during times of fatigue. In the next chapter, I discuss balancing the energy in times of increased inflammation, or "flares." The next section of the book continues through the subtler layers of the energy and mind as we continue relating yoga's PMK model to living with arthritis.

PART II

THRIVING WITH
ARTHRITIS

Part II of *Yoga* Therapy *for Arthritis* builds upon the physical and energetic experiences described and practiced in Part I. As we continue deepening the journey into the *pancamaya koshas* (PMK), or "layers" of a whole person, we inevitably arrive in more subtle realms. While the physical body and its energetic patterns are more obvious and changeable, our mental, psychological, and spiritual aspects are subtle. It takes quiet contemplation and gentle, sustained effort to change the way we think, feel, and simply "are" in the world. This part of the book brings you yoga and scientific theory and practice to connect a healthy mental state to a physical sense of wellbeing. More importantly, routines for daily life—and the beliefs that support them—are highlighted.

Chapter 6

ARTHRITIS AND ENERGY LEVELS

"Arthritis" may combine Latin *words* for joint and inflammation but not all of the many conditions under its banner are primarily conditions of joint inflammation. Most are, however. As mentioned previously, the most common arthritic condition, OA, was once thought to involve only localized swelling in the affected joint(s). It is now known that even OA involves some systemic inflammation, although to a lesser degree than other forms of arthritis, such as RA, gout, or psoriatic arthritis. Diseases of systemic inflammation and immune dysregulation often exhibit symptoms of fatigue, especially during flares, or exacerbations in disease activity. This chapter continues looking at PMK through the lens of lacking vitality. I discuss inflammation and other factors contributing to fatigue in arthritis and offer ways that yoga can support people during flares of heightened inflammation and symptom severity.

Complex Factors in Inflammatory Arthritis and Fatigue

Systemic arthritis conditions are diagnosed with three types of evaluation: physical assessment, patient report, and bloodwork. The physical assessment examines the joint, including tenderness and swelling, determines the degree of morning stiffness, and uses radiographs (x-rays) to assess connective tissue loss. The patient report includes questions about symptom characteristics, severity, and timing. The bloodwork measures inflammatory markers in the bloodstream. These markers include proteins that are released during an inflammatory response such as C-reactive protein and interleukin-6.

In systemic inflammation, white blood cells are released into the blood stream and travel to affected areas as part of an immune response. In an autoimmune process, the body has mistakenly identified some of its own tissue as foreign and is attacking that tissue as it would an invader such as a bacterial or viral infection. This process tends to result in redness, swelling, and pain. It is often accompanied by flu-like symptoms, such as fatigue, chills, fever, aches, loss of appetite, and a lack of clear-headedness. Fatigue can be further complicated by the common comorbid issues of obesity, sleep disturbance, and pain. The connections between these issues are complex.

Some of the complexities regarding obesity are that low activity due to arthritis pain and fatigue lead to obesity and obesity itself is a risk factor for OA. Since two-thirds of Americans are overweight or obese, many people living with arthritis carry excess body weight. This has an impact on joint structure, disease processes, and pain through the extra pressure and friction on the joints, particularly weight-bearing joints such as the knees and hips. Additionally, carrying extra weight can impact energy regardless of pain or other arthritis symptoms. Imagine putting on a 50-pound backpack before going out for your usual daily activities. The extra weight literally requires more energy to just carry it around. This is one of the reasons that people who lose weight report having more energy.

Obesity is also associated with sleep apnea and being overweight can make it difficult to be comfortable during sleep, both of which can also impact energy levels. As previously discussed, though, adipose tissue (fat) can be thought of as an active endocrine (hormonal) organ, not just inert tissue. Obesity is an inflammatory condition itself. Those inflammatory markers mean that all the pathways by which inflammation impacts energy can also be present for overweight individuals with less inflammatory arthritis. In fact, metabolic and psychological factors may explain the sleepiness associated with obesity more so than the resulting sleep apnea or sleep disturbances.[72]

Eighty percent of people living with arthritis, whether overweight or not, report some form of sleep disturbance. Sleep challenges among people with arthritis are complex and extend beyond the obvious sleep interference that may come from nighttime pain. People with arthritis may have sleep habits that result in poorer sleep, including daytime napping, irregular sleep schedules, and eating too much before bed. Some arthritis medications may also interfere with sleep,[73] and people lose sleep with anxiety, depression, or general worries about the impacts of arthritis on daily life.

Sleep issues are known to worsen pain. In fact, the relationship may be strongest in that direction. A study including people with OA showed that participants reported sleep disturbance regardless of their pain levels at bedtime, and a poor night's sleep predicted greater pain the next day.[74] Three-quarters of people with chronic pain also report fatigue and there is a correlation between pain severity and fatigue in arthritis.[75] This relationship can be cyclical and complicated, since fatigue also impacts the experience of pain and the capacity for coping. Diabetics with chronic pain were given a medication often used to treat nerve pain, which resulted in improvements in pain and pain's interference with sleep and vitality.[76] Complicating this even further, that medication is also used to treat depression and anxiety, both of which can impact pain, sleep, and fatigue. Interestingly, there may also be hormones involved in the relationship between pain and fatigue, which could be part of the reason that more women than men are impacted by pain/fatigue conditions such as fibromyalgia.[77]

This relationship between pain and fatigue is partly biological but may also be due to the overwhelming challenges of managing arthritis pain and disability. The dysregulation of the ANS and the stress response that is turned on by challenging circumstances may also be implicated in arthritis fatigue. There are also complex relationships within the hypothalamic-pituitary-adrenal (HPA) axis, which may be involved in sleep regulation, of course impacting energy and fatigue.[78] A heightened stress response can increase production of corticoids (steroid hormones), ultimately including glucocorticoid resistance and subsequent fatigue.[79] Living with a painful chronic disease in general can be overwhelming and tiring. Sara Nash, who shares her experience of life with RA in comics, once wrote a wanted ad asking for a superhero assistant to fulfill all of the roles and responsibilities that make RA a full-time job, on top of whatever other work and family demands life may carry. As we sometimes say, life with arthritis requires extra bandwidth, and coping with pain and its consequences is partly why. Unfortunately, fatigue can limit that very bandwidth and impede arthritis coping.

RA Is a Full-Time Job

Sara Nash, Yoga for Arthritis graduate and host of Single Gal's Guide to RA blog[80] writes about how living with arthritis is like another job. Not only does disease bring challenges like fatigue, weakness, and pain, but all other requirements that go into living with arthritis—appointments, injections, nutritional demands, physical therapies, etc.—add up on top of all life's normal responsibilities. Here is Sarah's story in her own words:

Getting diagnosed with a disease, especially a chronic one, means that you have a new, full time job—like it or not. It doesn't matter if you already have a full time job and are swamped, and it doesn't matter if you'll actually be good at this job, either. Once you qualify, it's yours. The benefits for this new job are lousy. There's no vacation (though you do get plenty of sick days, *har har har*), the hours are vicious and include weekends, evenings, and early mornings. There are no retirement benefits. You can't take a vacation. You not only *don't* get paid for this job, it actually costs you.

When I was first diagnosed with RA, I left my rheumatologist's office, where I had already scheduled a follow-up appointment in six weeks time, and went immediately next door to the ophthalmology department to make an appointment with a doctor there. I continued on to have chest x-rays for the cardiologist about my heart murmur. When I got back to my office for my *other* full time job, I called to schedule the appointment with the cardiologist and the neurologist (for migraines). In successive weeks, I would also have to schedule two additional appointments with the ophthalmologist, begin physical therapy sessions one to two times per week, and schedule an echocardiogram, an MRI, and more follow-up appointments. And there is always, always, always, more blood work. At times, I feel more like a pin cushion than a person.

To say that I felt overwhelmed would be like saying the Tour de France is a bit of a bike ride. I felt completely snowed under and unprepared. Honestly, how was I going to do all of this? I already had a ridiculously busy life filled with meetings, travel, going to performances, receptions, yoga, and squeezing in time with my friends. Now I was going to have to fit in all these other appointments and become the manager of a medical team—my medical team. No one could be a better manager or advocate for my own health than I would be. I had to remember when I was supposed to see whom, what had happened the last time, what I needed from which doctor, etc.

Luckily, organization has never been my weak point, so after I got over my initial phase of mind-numbing denial and panic, I went out, bought a cute little notebook and an expandable mini-file folder system and began keeping track of all my doctors, appointments, tests, medicines, blood pressure and other vitals, bills, insurance requests (and denials—blah), and receipts. For most of December, January, and February, I had between two and four appointments per week, every week. Thankfully, this new job is calming down for now. I've gotten the hang of it, partly, so I'm not as overwhelmed, and it's not quite so demanding. My physical therapy is winding down. The initial battery of tests is over, so I see my rheumatologist every six to eight weeks and all my other doctors every six months to a year. I am managing prescription refill schedules (I swear I am dropping one off or picking one up every time I turn around), insurance paperwork and staying on top of my preventative care with modalities like yoga and bodywork.

I hope I'm not up for any type of promotion at this new job. I am, for once, perfectly content and would prefer not to move up. I'm hoping if I play my cards right, I can stay in this lower management position for the rest of my days and not attract too much attention from the higher-ups. Who knows, with all the scientific and medical research being done, maybe one day I might actually get fired!

Is Fatigue Worse than Pain?

Sara's story illustrates some of the factors that make arthritis so mentally and physically fatiguing. Particularly in my experience working with individual clients, I have heard countless times that "the fatigue is worse than the pain." At first blush, this seems illogical—how can wanting to sleep possibly be the cause of more suffering than unrelenting physical pain? So, of course, I've asked that question of my clients with RA, lupus, and other systemic arthritis conditions. To understand it, you have to use a whole-person approach and think about the many aspects of life that are impacted by arthritis. You also have to consider the mind's remarkable ability to adapt to pain signalling. Let's start with the latter issue.

The reason for physical pain is to elicit a change in behavior. If you put your hand on a hot stove and feel pain, you will remove your hand from the stove quickly, thereby sparing more severe skin damage. In the case of chronic pain, the relationship between physical risk and pain severity becomes less aligned, and the pain is more strongly influenced by a variety of non-physical factors. In a condition like RA, where there can be a baseline of pain even in the absence of movement or pressure on the joints, it can feel as though the pain information is less useful and actionable. As a result, there can be a tendency to try to ignore it, or "push through it."

The concept of pushing through pain is about shutting off attention to the physical experience and this disconnect between mind and body is a common coping strategy in the face of chronic pain. However, it is much harder to push through fatigue. For anyone who has suffered a terrible flu or lived through early pregnancy or early parenting, you can probably relate to this. There are times that the body just feels incapacitated and refuses to cooperate with whatever plans we have in mind. We might even fall asleep against our will. While pain interferes with work, relationships, and other commitments, fatigue may interfere even more. This notion is also born out in the research literature, where fatigue is discussed by patients as a prominent and important feature of RA flares.[81]

There are a variety of mechanisms to explain why heightened disease activity in rheumatic diseases is associated with fatigue. It makes sense that when the immune system is mounting a response, fatigue, would result from diverting energy and resources away from normal biological functions and toward immune function. This may partly explain the fatigue associated with many illnesses that require an immune response, such as a viral or bacterial infection. Additionally, inflammatory markers have been implicated in fatigue, and treatments that work by reducing inflammatory cytokines are effective in improving fatigue.[82] Elevated inflammatory markers can also result in anemia by decreasing iron levels,[83] which, in turn, causes fatigue due to a lack of oxygenated blood.

There may even be a direct effect of inflammation on the brain, despite the general protection of the brain from inflammatory processes. Following organ inflammation, specific pro-inflammatory cytokines are able to enter the brain in some areas with higher permeability of the blood-brain barrier,[84] and several animal studies demonstrate that the brain also produces cytokines which may be implicated in fatigue.[85]

While there appear to be many ways in which inflammation and fatigue may be related, there is no question that fatigue is a central symptom of inflammatory arthritis and must be considered in disease management, self-care, work-life balance, and yoga practice. Some forms of arthritis are autoimmune conditions that have high levels of systemic inflammation, but fatigue has BPSS causes and effects and may be experienced by those with other forms of arthritis for a variety of reasons also.

Yoga for Arthritis Fatigue

We know that yoga has an impact on the experience of arthritis symptoms, but it is not yet known whether yoga changes the underlying disease activity of inflammatory arthritis. In our research at Johns Hopkins,[86] there was a significant decrease in the number of tender and swollen joints for participants with RA. This suggests that disease activity may have decreased. However, there was also a decrease in the number of tender and swollen joints for the control group that did not quite reach statistical significance. A preliminary report of our findings did uncover a statistically significant change in the Disease Activity Score (DAS), which includes the number of tender and swollen joints along with a marker of systemic inflammation (the erythrocyte sedimentation rate or C-reactive protein) and a patient assessment of disease activity.[87] Another eight-week yoga program also reported statistically significant changes in DAS between the yoga and control groups.[88] Some studies have measured ring size as a marker of inflammation in the hands, although results have been mixed.[89] A randomized controlled trial published in 2011 that included 40 days of daily yoga[90] found significant reduction in stiffness, lymphocyte count (white blood cells) and uric acid, which is implicated in gout. However, they did not see a difference between the yoga and control groups for the number of inflamed joints and C-reactive protein, an inflammatory marker.

The randomized controlled trials in yoga tend to have small sample sizes, and larger studies are needed for more conclusive findings about the role of yoga in affecting the underlying inflammatory processes of arthritic conditions. The effects of yoga on inflammation in other conditions (stress, hypertension, cancer, heart disease) has been explored, and findings for these populations are also mixed, likely for similar reasons. Thus, we are uncertain whether yoga benefits the underlying inflammatory disease process. Future research should aim to determine this relationship more definitively.

There is good reason to believe yoga benefits symptoms and manifestations of the disease process, including fatigue. Vitality, or energy, was the outcome measure from our research most related to fatigue. For participants with RA or OA who received an eight-week yoga program of twice weekly group classes and weekly home practice, vitality improved by almost 30 per cent. This improvement persisted even nine months later, when we invited participants back for follow-up testing. It is important to consider that participants in our research had stable, well-managed disease that did not exhibit frequent flares. This suggests that yoga may improve energy for people living with arthritis, but we don't know what the effect would be for people in an active arthritis flare. Other studies have measured fatigue more directly and have also found improvements in RA fatigue associated with yoga practice.[91] In our qualitative research, minority participants with RA and OA reported feeling more energy and less fatigue after yoga classes.[92] Additional studies are needed to determine the specific effects of various yoga practices in the face of the fatigue experienced in active arthritis flares.

A Different Kind of Calculus

If you have ever tried to explain the impacts of your fatigue to loved ones, you know how hard it can be for others to understand. Low energy is debilitating. We only have so many resources to allocate to the many, many tasks of everyday life.

Healthy people do not measure the resources it takes to meet their basic physical needs. Everyday tasks are performed without much thought and without a sense that they are draining energy. Where the average person starts the day and arrives at work prepared to face the obligations, someone suffering from fatigue may have used up all their resources before getting to work!

People living with fatigue don't haphazardly go through their daily activities. Every action is measured because everything that isn't rest draws from highly limited resources. People living with inflammatory disease wake up with less energy, and some days there are fewer resources available than others. There is not enough energy to do all of the small daily requirements such as shower, prepare food, clean the house, care for children, and so on. All parts of daily life use resources; therefore, they must make critical choices about what is essential and what can be discarded. This is a different kind of calculus to regulate daily choices. It is important to pay attention to what is nourishing and what is draining…and eliminate as much of the latter as possible. Even simple things matter that might not even register as decisions for healthy people, like whether to wash their hair in the shower or to stand in the train. You can sometimes borrow from tomorrow's resources, but then you will wake up with even fewer the next day.

Your friends may wonder how you can possibly live like this every day. The recommendation is to be prepared for the unexpected. Never let your resources get down to zero. While this might mean cancelling plans or changing obligations, it allows there to be an energy reserve. Life with systemic arthritis means always being aware of how much energy you have and using it deliberately.

In time, some people even see this is a blessing. It means never wasting time or energy on something that doesn't matter. So…what are you doing with your resources each day? As Mary Oliver asked, "What will you do with your one wild and precious life?"

Yoga for Flares

While fatigue often occurs during inflammatory arthritis flares and requires more rest and possible changes in medical management, fatigue can also occur outside the context of an arthritis flare. Everyone experiences fatigue sometimes, having nothing to do with underlying disease processes, and this is also true for people living with arthritis. It is important to identify whether fatigue is an arthritis symptom or not. For some, the fatigue of arthritis might feel very different in its characteristics and severity. If this is not the case, consider any other arthritis symptoms that may be present.

Another consideration is whether the fatigue is happening after routine daily activities or whether another explanation is apparent. If the fatigue is unrelated to arthritis, there are other yoga practices that might help to energize the body and mind, providing greater mental clarity and capacity to fulfill the day's tasks and demands. Anyone who is uncertain whether their fatigue is arthritis-related might consider speaking to a medical doctor or rheumatology nurse in more detail to learn more.

It is critical to speak with a rheumatologist at the first sign of a flare. He or she might prescribe fast-acting medication to address the flare and can make recommendations about how to modify a yoga practice based on specific disease characteristics. Cancelling plans may be warranted when possible to allow for more rest. Similarly, communication with loved ones is key. Someone in a flare might consider asking for extra help and letting them know about the need for increased self-care. Nourishing and easily digested foods may also be in order. By managing energy in this way, it may be possible to shorten the duration or severity of the flare.

Once the proper external provisions (medical care, simplifying commitments, finding extra time for rest, etc.) are in place, consider the content and quality of an appropriate yoga practice. No matter the level of fatigue, it is always possible to practice yoga. If you have a mind and a body, you can practice yoga. It is also important that the yoga practice fits the current state of mind and body without doing harm. During mild fatigue, a gently physical practice and breathing techniques may be appropriate. Movement can still be beneficial, but should be modified to be slower, gentler, and done with support. During extreme fatigue, restorative poses in bed may be all that is possible or warranted. I have a student who was meditating while lying in bed during flares before she even knew what meditation was. I tell clients and students that pushing through fatigue is not only futile, but counter-productive. The body is suggesting a slowing down. It needs to rest.

Because a flare involves heightened inflammation, it is generally a good idea to avoid yoga practices that might be aggravating, excessively rigorous, or stressful to the joints. This includes poses that generate heat in the body, such as hot yoga, power yoga, fast-paced advanced classes, inversions and deep backbends that raise blood pressure (headstand, shoulderstand, camel, etc.), and strenuous breathing practices such as breath of fire (*kapalabhati*). Avoid poses that apply excess body weight and pressure to any affected joints, which will differ for each individual. A flare is a state of overactive immune activation involving heat and inflammation, so yoga practices should focus on fostering a state of calm and cooling.

It may also be beneficial to consider practices that can help to address fatigue. Depending on the severity of the flare and its unique characteristics, this might take a lot of different forms. In the case of a minor uptick in symptom severity, a gentle *asana* practice with slow-moving sequences, shorter holds, and lots of breath integration might be helpful. A therapeutic, gentle or restorative class might be available. At the very least, someone experiencing a flare or other fatigue should let their yoga teacher know that a gentler, modified practice might be warranted. Someone attending a yoga class should always feel free to modify the practice in any way that feels appropriate. Even resting in a relaxation posture and envisioning oneself performing the *asanas* has beneficial effects on the body, mind, and energy.

Sometimes sleep itself is the best form of practice. A short, guided meditation via recording or live instruction might be easier to sustain than a longer self-guided one. Slow, cooling breath such as the *sheetali pranayama* from Chapter 10 might be considered. For someone in a more severe flare, restorative poses in bed, recorded or live yoga nidra, sleep, and solitude might be more appropriate. Remember, there is a difference between choosing practices to combat fatigue, like those in the previous chapter, and practices that are modified to accommodate fatigue. The following practices are recommended during flares. They allow the restorative benefits of yoga with minimal risk of exacerbating inflammatory response and other symptoms.

Yoga Practice Is a State of Mind

Yoga's concepts of mindfulness and non-grasping (*aparighraha*) are critical to the use of yoga in the face of rheumatic fatigue. Mindfulness allows us to notice what is happening in our current experience on all *kosha* levels. It prevents us from being taken by surprise with a severe flare and overwhelming fatigue, because we have begun to notice the whisper that precedes the scream. Once this has been noticed, then the hard work of not grasping, or wanting the situation to be any different, begins.

The ability to witness our thoughts, feelings, sensations, and other internal cues are key to the practice of mindfulness. We can apply mindful awareness to our physical cues, as well. As we come to learn about individual manifestations of inflammation, pain, and the many lifestyle considerations, sensitivity increases regarding the early warning signs of a flare. Some people living with arthritis and related conditions may be surprised by their ability to intervene and reduce flare severity or duration.

It is also ideal to recuperate in small bits. Even if life requires continued work, caring for small children, or a large list of demands, there are still moments to recharge. Even a minute or two of relaxation, or a single deep breath, recruit the body's healing resources and bring some enlivenment back to the system. Remaining mindful of one's needs in the moment, without wishing things were different, fosters greater appreciation for the details of a good life, which can help to reduce suffering and malcontent.

Remember that different people have different phrasing for exertion and recovery. Pay attention to how you or your clients need to recuperate, and honor that method. You may notice that the body prefers brief periods of exertion and then requires brief recuperative periods. Alternatively, exertion may occur for extended periods, with mindful awareness regarding bodily messages and arising thoughts, followed by a more prolonged rest. If you wait until the body forces recuperation, it will be longer and more extreme, often with worse symptoms; therefore, it is important to trust signals and cues while practicing mindfulness. While not necessarily easy, it is a yoga practice to work toward accepting those cues without grasping for a different body, energy level, or symptom set. You might be surprised at the benefits that arise from such a practice.

POSTURE: BED YOGA

Years ago, Nancy O'Brien, a person with arthritis, was in search of a more integrative approach. She experienced challenges with her medical care and complications from surgery, including a two-and-a-half-month hospital stay and time spent in a coma! An integrative doctor connected her with the Integral Yoga community, some of whom were working in a hospital-based yoga program. After an initial visit at the hospital, Nancy was then visited by a yoga teacher one or two times per week. She was hardly able to sit or stand due to organ challenges and lack of muscular support, so her entire yoga practice had to be done lying down.

Nancy is now an active, thriving yoga teacher and therapist, among the first group to be trained in the Yoga for Arthritis program, and the matriarch of New York City's vibrant Yoga for Arthritis and Chronic Pain *sangha* (community). She still practices yoga in her bed as a key component of her self-care, and shares some of her experiences and recommendations here.

During some of her most debilitating times, Nancy's yoga practice would start with grounding through her feet, using the wall, foot board, or yoga blocks, and working up through the body, integrating with her breath. She would align herself as she was working up through the body, supported by the bed, but energized in all directions. One of her favorite poses became reclining Tree Pose. It gave her so much hope and strength to be able to get into that pose when she was unable to serve in her roles as wife, mother, and professional in the ways she had previously. She felt so vital in her practice; it allowed her to change her relationship to her body, the pain, and the debilitation she was experiencing. Tree pose was really an epiphany—that she could have this much energy and engagement lying down. Through that pose, she felt a sense of balance, strength, and hope.

Eventually, her yoga practice helped her to become stronger and more capable, but also more resilient and hopeful. It opened a new doorway to affirmation, meditation, and sometimes just moving her fingers and toes in response to her body's needs. Parts of her body hurt just from laying there, so being able to engage muscles and do so much with intention really changed her experience. If her back hurt, she could lower and raise her tailbone just a bit. She would think of areas of pain or *dukha* (suffering) and focus on a word, like courage, while breathing into that area of the body. She continued to be guided through these practices by Integral Yoga teachers during the nearly two years that she was out of work. Small actions had a large impact and she was gradually able to do more.

Nancy recalls that she would meet herself exactly where she was on any given day, with no expectations of continuing to improve. This required a great deal of compassion. She shared with me that she would like the following embroidered on a pillow to remind her: "Meet yourself exactly where you are at this moment, with compassion." Like many people with arthritis, her recovery was not a straight line of improvement, but more of a roller-coaster. This perspective of equanimity helped to keep her from despairing over the lack of progress, so that any "goals" became irrelevant. Her yoga practice wasn't about trying to be more able, just about feeling better now. This experience also allows her to better understand the challenges of living with a chronic disabling condition such as arthritis, where reversal of disease progression may not be possible, but feeling better most certainly is. Eventually, Nancy worked with her yoga teachers to build strength and function.

Here are Nancy's recommendations for a "bed yoga" practice, incorporating forward bend, backbend, side bend, and twist postures.

As soon as consciousness comes, and sometimes that means being awakened from sleep by pain or discomfort, start with a focus on gratitude. This allows a shift out of any fear, anger, or resentment that might arise.

From a place of gratitude, start engaging the body with Three-Part Breath (see Chapter 3), focusing especially on mindful exhalations.

A side stretch is often the easiest way to begin movement, because it opens everything up and allows for fuller breath. Slide one limb at a time over to the same side, moving one leg, then the other, one arm, then the other. Feel a slow, gentle opening and breathe into that space.

For a forward bend, lift one or both knees to the chest, circling the knees as if drawing circles on the ceiling above. This might also lead to other leg movements, like sliding the heels along the bed, coordinated with the breath.

To twist, bend one knee in toward the chest, or place the foot flat on the bed. Allow that knee to fall over to the opposite side. Alternately, let both knees fall to one side, or slide them up into a fetal position, rolling the torso open to face the ceiling. Consider supporting the knees with blankets or pillow to allow release and relaxation. Think of the twist as an exploration. Where is there unnecessary holding? Back off, breathe in, and notice if deepening becomes available. Think of the twist as being internal, and not about whatever shape the body might be making.

Moving into backbend, gently roll over onto the belly or side. If lying on your belly, place hands or a pillow under the forehead so that the chin can be slightly tucked and cervical spine elongated. The arms may also rest alongside the body. Curl the toes under and reach through the back of the heels. If possible, lift the heel, allowing the toes to relax. You can also use the end of the bed to lengthen by placing the feet over the end of the bed and using that to stabilize, drawing the toes toward the belly and perhaps lifting one leg. If lying on one side, bend the top knee, reaching the heel toward the tailbone. Draw the shoulders back and open the chest. You might even be able to reach the foot, and press the foot into the hand.

From here, consider trying reclining Tree Pose. Roll onto the back, pressing a foot into the footboard, wall, or a yoga block. Lengthen through the spine, finding alignment in each part of the body from toes to crown of head. Feel the stability, grounding, and power of the pose.

Allow the body to rest into *Savasana*, perhaps with pillows under the knees, head, or anywhere else that needs support. Move through a progressive relaxation in your mind, with a teaching, or via a recording. This might even be followed by a meditation of your choice.

This sequence, or any part of it, can be performed in the middle of the night if you can't sleep! Eventually, you may be able to sit on side of bed and move into Cat-Cow, a seated forward bend, seated spinal twist and even a supported back bend with pillows behind you. After some seated movements, you might be able to rise into Mountain, bringing hands to heart and set an intention for your day. This is a full yoga practice before even going to the bathroom!

For Nancy, yoga wasn't an isolated practice, but an ongoing way of responding to her body's needs. She now feels that her ongoing recovery is enabled by "doing yoga" 24–7. This allows her to function. If she didn't do it, she would be so deconditioned that she would not be able to move through her life as she does. She notices that she is constantly suffusing energy into areas that are blocked off. It is a kind of constant monitoring of pain, weakness, and energy, responding to those needs in the moment. This experience has provided her with a deeper sense of appreciation for anyone on the street in New York City with cane or walker. She recognized that it probably took them hours to get out of bed. Other people around them may be frustrated because they are moving slowly and Nancy just marvels at them and thinks "Yay you!"

Summary

This chapter relates PMK, the energy layer, to coping with the low energy often associated with inflammation and arthritis. Fatigue is a part of modern life and is especially debilitating for people with systemic forms of arthritis, such as RA. Obesity, low activity, and sleep issues are also factors. Even in times of debilitating fatigue, there are still yoga practices that can be performed to enhance mobility and maintain peace of mind and a sense of self. Great care is required during flares and it is beneficial to remain aware of early warning signs in order to intervene before the symptoms become overwhelming. Carry the mindfulness from yoga into life to gain everyday enjoyment and become more discerning about how to expend energy and when to rest. The following chapter looks at the common arthritis symptom of pain and how the mind, *manomaya kosha*, plays a role in coping.

Chapter 7

PAIN IN THE BRAIN (*MANOMAYA KOSHA*)

Yoga offers many strategies for coping with pain. As we learn more about the neurobiology of pain and the effects of arthritis on the brain and central nervous system (CNS), there is greater evidence for the benefits of yoga on arthritis. The mind, *manomaya kosha*, plays a role in the perception and experience of pain. In osteoporosis, for example, there is sometimes little relationship between arthritis severity and arthritis pain. In other words, some people have severe tissue damage but minimal pain, while others have mild damage and overwhelming pain. Because of this, there is an opportunity to impact pain, even if the tissue damage remains. Therefore, patients should be in ongoing dialog with medical and complementary care providers about the best combination of approaches for arthritis management in all of its stages. In this chapter, I will discuss the multiple factors influencing pain and how yoga relaxation, conscious movement, and meditation impact thought, emotion, and psychology. Healthcare workers and people with arthritis can apply a variety of yoga methods and philosophy to help cope with and transcend the symptoms of the disease.

Pain and Healthcare

I often tell people that they are the world's leading expert of their own bodies. I also reinforce that each individual should have the right to autonomous decision-making (when possible) about their own health choices. Ideally, each person is able to make those decisions with access to the information necessary to guide those decisions. For example, you have the right to smoke cigarettes but you should make that decision understanding the health risks associated with such behavior. Similarly, people living with chronic disease can choose to pursue whatever health treatments they choose from among the available options. In order to do that with sufficient information, however, it is always advisable to seek medical supervision and guidance. I know that many people turn to complementary therapies because the medical care or guidance they have received seems underwhelming or inadequate. I also know people whose lives are transformed by their relationship with a medical provider.

Just as you shop around before making a major purchase, so should you feel justified, even obligated, in exploring medical providers in your area. If you don't feel heard by your doctor, if you don't feel comfortable with the communication, style, or approach that your doctor takes, you might consider other options. You should have a doctor you trust—a doctor who will be a partner in your health journey.

Additionally, there is no harm in getting information and answers to your questions, even seeking more than one perspective. Doctors are very accustomed to the process of second opinions and your doctor is unlikely to be offended when/if you decide to get another perspective to inform your medical decisions. In fact, I know of situations where a doctor has encouraged second opinions and looks forward to learning about their colleagues' perspective about a situation or treatment decision. Be sure to approach medical visits with an open mind and a willingness to truly hear the reasoning behind your doctor's recommendations. Ultimately, of course, the choice about how to proceed is yours.

For optimal healthcare, communicate with your medical providers about any complementary therapies you are using or considering, including yoga. Some therapies interact, like herbs and medication, so it is important to discuss those choices with all of your providers.

Sometimes, people living with pain conditions feel as though their symptoms and concerns are not taken seriously by medical providers, which may lead them to seek other approaches to care. While medicine has made impressive advancements in the management of many conditions, including autoimmune diseases, the management of chronic pain remains a challenge. Some pain conditions have been historically misunderstood and disregarded as psychologically based without any physiological basis. While we know that psychological stress and mood most certainly impact pain and other disease symptoms, conditions such as fibromyalgia (FM) and chronic fatigue can also be explained physiologically. It is therefore wise to manage both the physiological and psychological processes that are part of the disease.

Often, providers of complementary care are able to take more time with each patient and operate from a whole-person perspective, which can be better suited to complex BPSS conditions than a systems-based approach. Ideally, someone living with a challenging chronic condition is able to find the combination of a sympathetic, compassionate, patient medical provider and the most appropriate self-care and complementary approaches for optimizing health outcomes and quality of life.

Pain in the Brain

Acute pain, that which is immediate and has an end, is different from chronic pain, which can last a lifetime at varying intensities. While acute pain in some situations does not even involve the brain, registering only in the spinal cord for greater efficiency (i.e. hand on a hot stove), chronic pain is closely tied to the workings of the brain itself. In fact, our thoughts and feelings have a remarkably powerful impact on the perception of pain. As the duration of pain increases from acute to chronic (greater than three months), there is a less direct relationship between tissue damage and pain. Instead, the influences on pain severity are much more influenced by cognitive and emotional factors. In knee OA, for example, there are some individuals with mild disease and high levels of pain, whereas others have more progressed arthritis but very little pain.[93] While it may not immediately seem so, this is very good news. People don't get joint replacements because their arthritis has progressed. They get surgery because the arthritis symptoms are interfering with their quality of life and daily activities. Since arthritis cannot be reversed at the level of the joint, we can instead turn to the workings of the brain to impact pain levels.

While the workings of the brain affect our experience of pain, surprisingly the reverse is also true. Chronic pain can change the anatomy and function of brain circuitry. In fact, the same brain functions that most impact pain levels (descending pain modulatory systems) are the ones that are changed by pain itself.[94] This creates a negative feedback loop whereby pain changes brain and brain changes pain. The result is increased pain and increased mental and emotional comorbidities often seen in chronic pain populations (mental fog, depressive symptoms, etc.). These increases in pain and associated symptoms happen regardless of the actual challenges of living with the disease that can impact mental/emotional states more directly.

An important region of the brain for pain regulation is the anterior cingulate cortex (ACC), which has been considered part of the emotional brain. Those with damage to the ACC have changes in their emotional response to pain. This region of the brain can be activated without any tissue damage, simply by observing another individual in pain.[95] Interestingly, research has shown that people can learn to control the activity in their ACC through cognitive strategies.[96] The more control they develop, the less pain they feel when faced with an experimental pain stimulus. This means that we can learn to control the parts of our brain that hold the dial on pain intensity. In fact, negative emotions evoked by experiences like emotional faces, unpleasant music, or strong odors can change several regions of the brain related to pain, including the ACC. However, positive experiences and expectations can provide pain relief. Placebo pain medication (sugar pill) changes opioid activity in the ACC, as well as other brain regions.[97] Therefore, someone using medication may have more or less of a response depending on their emotional state and/or expectations of the medicine's effect.

What I find especially fascinating and critically important for people with arthritis is that chronic pain changes the experience of all other painful stimuli. When people with knee arthritis put their hands in an ice bath, for example, the hand discomfort is stronger than if they didn't have knee pain. Even stimuli that are not painful for healthy adults may feel painful for those with chronic pain, due to overactivation of certain brain pathways.[98] Fortunately, this can be reversed. When a painful condition is eliminated, the grey matter associated with chronic pain is returned to normal size. In other words, pain reduces grey matter, and once the pain is eliminated, grey matter expands.

We also know that meditation thickens grey matter in these brain regions, including the ACC, insula, and pre-frontal cortex.[99] Therefore, the impact of chronic pain on the brain may be reversed or prevented with the practice of meditation. While most people think of *asana* practice as most important for managing arthritis, the relevance of meditation for chronic pain management should not be overlooked. In other words, don't skip the meditation. It might actually be the most helpful aspect of yoga practice! On days when an *asana* practice seems overwhelming or inaccessible, consider turning to the yoga practices of the mind.

While changes in brain structure are powerful, the context and meaning of pain help to explain enormous variations in individual pain experiences. The stories we have about our pain—what it means, how it will change our life, what we can expect—help to dictate the pain we experience. Although the mechanisms differ, pain in both OA and RA are influenced by stress,[100] and higher levels of pain are reported on days of greater stress. Therapies that focus on stress reduction show decreased pain, supporting the connection between stress and symptoms.[101] While meditation practices allow us the space to choose dispassion regarding our circumstances, yoga philosophy can also help to shape our relationship to disease and therefore our experience of it. Practicing the yoga ethics of contentment (*santosha*) and non-grasping (*aparigraha*), for example, may help to ameliorate some of the negative loops of pain, cognition, and emotion that render arthritis so incapacitating.

It is easy to say that we can change our brains, choose to be unflappable and avoid the story associated with the pain. In truth, these are monumental tasks. They require long-term commitment and challenging effort for perhaps inconsistent and unpredictable results. Just as it isn't easy to get on a yoga mat every morning, it also isn't easy to find contentment in the most overwhelming circumstances or to clear the mind when the body is exhausted. Judging self or others on account of the relationships between pain, cognition, and emotion is neither fair nor productive. It is important to remember, however, that the solutions for arthritis management are not all in the cartilage, and that many tools of yoga can be harnessed to help improve quality of life for those suffering from arthritis symptoms.

Fibromyalgia: Is the Pain "All in Your Head"?

FM has a challenging history as a diagnosis. The problem mainly stems from the fact that FM was misunderstood by the medical community for many years. FM patients are often treated by rheumatologists, even though it is not an autoimmune condition, like RA or lupus, nor is it a joint condition, like OA or gout. (Some people with clinical evidence of arthritis also meet criteria for having fibromyalgia.) Because of that, if a doctor were to run the standard blood tests that are used to diagnose many rheumatic diseases, they might not show anything noteworthy. Similarly, an image of the joints via x-ray or MRI might show nothing, even in the places of greatest pain.

As a result, many doctors came to the conclusion that FM was a psychosomatic condition in which an emotional disturbance of some kind was causing patients to experience pain. Some medical professionals concluded that patients were perhaps exaggerating symptoms for attention-seeking or other psychological reasons. Unlike other conditions they treated, FM was difficult to understand and difficult to treat. FM is characterized by overactive pain pathways. There are no visible signs, but there are certain places in the body that are tender to touch and/or movement. It also differs from arthritis because the pain is not necessarily in the joints, but in a series of other points on the body. Some doctors would even suggest that "it is all in your head." And perversely, that is actually true!

FM is a CNS pain-processing disorder. Where is the central nervous system? That's right. It's in your head! (Well, your head and also the spinal cord.) The reason FM does not show up on x-rays and blood tests is that doctors were looking in the wrong place. FM is not in the joints and it doesn't share the same biomarkers as autoimmune conditions like RA. Of course, that doesn't make it any less real. The pain is absolutely real, as is the fatigue, the foggy-headedness, the memory challenges, and other symptoms. People with FM experience pain differently, due to the way that the nervous system is sensing, interpreting, and responding to stimuli. They even have higher levels of something called "substance P," which is related to the transmission of pain signals to the CNS, as well as different cytokine levels than people without FM.[102]

As for the psychology of it, we absolutely know that mood affects pain, and vice versa. So, it isn't surprising that people with FM often also have mood disorders. Again, that doesn't make the pain any less real. However, when it comes to treating FM, it's trickier because the mechanisms are different than for other pain conditions and a standard NSAID medication is unlikely to fully address the symptoms.

When considering a yoga practice, the challenges and opportunities for FM patients are also different. While there are specific "trigger points" that might be especially painful for people with FM, there is often a general sensitivity to any tactile stimuli. That means that the pressure of one body part on another, a surface like the floor, or a prop can be sources of pain.

Any additional difference is that, because there isn't necessarily joint damage (unless they also have arthritis, which is common), there may be less risk when choosing to stay with the discomfort and breathe into sensation. Of course, it is always ideal to speak with a trusted medical provider about any movements that should be avoided.

Because FM has been historically misunderstood, many people living with FM are tired of not being taken seriously, of fighting to get a proper diagnosis, of fiercely advocating for their own care, and of being rejected by some medical providers. Since we know that all of these experiences can impact the functioning of the CNS, listening attentively with loving kindness and compassion might have as much impact on symptoms as the breathing and movement practices themselves. This is where yoga teachers and therapists, as well as other health professionals, can have a strong positive impact. While it might be uncomfortable to sit in meditation for long durations, finding ways to infuse daily life with mindfulness, deep breathing and other self-care will be particularly important for improved CNS regulation, along with behavioral strategies such as sleep hygiene and management of external stimuli.

Placebo Knee Surgery

In 2013, results of a groundbreaking study were published. Some people with meniscal tears (but not OA), received knee surgery and others received mock surgery. Surprisingly, there was no difference in any primary outcomes when comparing surgery to placebo (mock surgery).[103] In fact, further follow-up demonstrated that two years later, there was still no difference between groups.[104] In other words, surgery for meniscal tears doesn't work. Or…does it?

To make sense of this study's findings, it is important to understand the concept of "non-specific effects" or "context effects," also referred to as placebo effects. When conducting research using models that have emerged in Western medical science, a placebo treatment is often used to differentiate the "specific" effects of the treatment (i.e. medication) from the effects of everything else involved in the treatment (patient–provider interaction, expectations, ritual, etc.). The reason this needs to be considered in research is that these other aspects of a treatment happen to be incredibly powerful! You might think of the placebo effect in medical research as the impact of the mind on the experience of the body. We also know that the size, color, smell, and form of a medicine all impact its effects. In some cases, the non-specific effects are so powerful that they are no different from the effects of the actual medication, or in this case, surgery. Surgery is poised to have a powerful effect because expectations are often high and there is actually a fair amount of ritual involved in the practice of medicine. Of course, we don't want to perform mock surgeries and subject patients to unnecessary risk, but the placebo effect is a real effect and it is helpful to consider how that can be harnessed in safe ways.

In fact, many integrative health practices are well-situated to optimize non-specific effects through greater attention to the patient–provider relationship, the creation of healing environments and the use of ritual.[105] Instead of considering these effects to be "fake" or "sham," it may serve us to optimize these effects. Combining non-specific effects *with* specific effects is the best formula for maximum impact. Integrating the best of what medicine has to offer (pharmacology and surgery) with the best of what complementary practices have to offer (relationship, environment, ritual) is in the best interest of patients who are interested and willing.

This is not to suggest that all of the effects of complementary practices are placebo. In fact, randomized controlled trials often find differences between treatment and placebo groups for such modalities. It is also often challenging to provide an adequate control group for such practices, since you can provide a fake medicine much more easily than a fake meditation. Similarly, most surgeries are not equal to their placebos. While surgery may not be more effective than placebo for meniscal tears, it *is* effective for treatment of OA. In fact, successful knee replacement surgery fosters the reversal of brain changes that occur as a result of chronic pain.[106]

Pain and the Eight-Fold Path of Yoga

All eight limbs of yoga—restraints, observances, physical practices, breathing exercises, sense mastery, concentration, meditation, and higher perspectives—can be applied to help work with the pain of arthritis. Each of these limbs contributes to an internal state, directing focus, and altering psychology and physiology for profound outcomes through all levels of a whole person. While, at first, these may not seem compelling, as people cultivate an established yoga practice and gain experience with its rich and subtle effects, these can become powerful tools for uplifting life and changing one's relationship with arthritis.

The restraints (*yamas*)—non-harm, truthfulness, proper direction of energy, non-stealing, and non-grasping—offer perspectives that support pain relief. Above all, do no harm. This means listening to the body and respecting the messages of pain, adapting when needed. Furthermore, it means not harming oneself with the "story" about the pain—all the fear and projections about what the pain means and how awful it makes things. Even though that may be true, it causes harm to ruminate in negative storylines. The truth of the story is that pain is present with a disease like arthritis; there are ways it can be shifted and there are some things about it that are outside of your personal control. Do not waste energy on worry, anger, fear, frustration, despair, and all the other normal but harmful emotions that go along with this. These emotions can be processed with a mental health professional to avoid both suppression and rumination. It is a waste to grasp for that which once was, or what we wish would be. Rather, follow the observances to gain more of what is truly desired—peace of mind and lightness of heart.

The *niyamas* teach the observance of healthy, balancing behaviors. Purity, contentment, effort/discipline, self-study, and surrender to the great unknown make up these five ethical principles. The intention towards internal and external health and purity guides us to make small but significant choices every day. For example, the routine of snacking on veggies and hummus will impact systemic health differently than low-nutrition snacks. Finding a way to be content with things as they are cultivates a deep inner peace and, as discussed above, may actually alter pain perception. Taking action on one's own behalf to create healthy routines, at whatever level of engagement is possible at that time, establishes a rhythm of self-care which becomes a habit. Once discipline is a habit, it seems to take care of itself most days. Learning about ourselves through research, spirituality, expression, and personal exploration all help integrate the realities of arthritis and set conditions for greater peace of mind.

The first two limbs provide context for the other six. The third limb of *asana*, which includes physical postures, relaxation, and hygiene, guides people with arthritis to move, rest, and care for the body. Various lifestyle practices like stretching, strengthening, progressive muscle relaxation, nutrition, hydration, and countless other physical care regimens all support the body in coping with and easing arthritis symptoms.

The fourth limb of breathing and energy practices (*pranayama*) may have an immediate and noticeable effect on symptoms like pain, fatigue, depression, and anxiety. Various techniques are available to up-regulate or down-regulate the nervous system, soothe emotions, enliven energy, and focus the mind.

The latter limbs of the eight-fold path are subtle as they move into the workings of the mind, physiological states and spiritual connections. *Pratyahara*, or sense mastery, teaches about the influence our senses have on our state of mind as we witness the relationship between the senses and the outer world and eventually, the relationship between sensory information and thought patterns. Once we are able to steady the senses, concentration and meditation are possible.

Concentration (*dharana*), what most modern society thinks of as meditation, is single-pointed focus. By holding the mind on a single concept, image, feeling, etc.— or, more accurately, by committing to call the mind back every time it wanders, which will be about once per second at first—the mind learns to stay focused. When one holds the mind single-pointedly for a period of time, consciousness shifts to a state of meditation (*dhyana*). Brainwaves change from beta to alpha or even theta, neural activity moves from frontal to central regions and there may arise a sense of timelessness or deep peace and clarity.

Enlightenment, union, or what is known in Sanskrit as *Samadhi* is a continuous state of wellbeing and connection. This pervasive sense of ease exists, even if a person is physically unwell or tragedies occur in life. There are many levels of *Samadhi*; they all involve presence and an accepting, peaceful perspective on life. This perspective is cultivated by living, thinking, and feeling in alignment with the ten ethical principles of yoga. You see, the yoga journey is synergistic and although there are progressive stages, all eight limbs are equally important and practiced together. You may think of the journey as a spiral, rather than a line.

Yoga Meditation and Pain

When a person with arthritis applies the sixth limb of concentration, there is an opportunity to shift the relationship with and even perception of chronic pain. One is able to discern between the objective experience of pain and the beliefs, or story. Hopes and fears, preconceived ideas, past experiences, personality, wants, wishes, and desires—all of those mental habits are more malleable than tissue pathology.

As mentioned earlier, there is compelling evidence that meditation is the most powerful of all yoga interventions for arthritis. (Remember, meditation is about the state of mind, not the position of the body.) The previous limbs of yoga set suitable conditions for meditation. While it takes patience and commitment to establish a meditation practice, the outcomes are worth it!

There are many different ways to meditate. Many people meditate while sitting on the floor, a cushion, or a bench. It can also be done sitting in a chair or standing. While lying down is often discouraged because of the tendency to fall asleep, I believe that meditating lying down is better than not meditating. In fact, I know some people who lie in bed and meditate for very long periods during an arthritis flare when not much else is possible. If you find that you are falling asleep during meditation, which can also happen while sitting up, consider whether the body needs rest more than the mind needs meditation, and try to meditate when you are fully rested, if possible. There are also moving meditations you might try that don't require being still.

In this chapter, you can use the Meditation Practices Sampler to explore various approaches to meditation and find what resonates with you. Once you have chosen an approach, commit to trying it with consistency for a while to see what happens. It is important to avoid self-judgment during meditation practice. There isn't anything in particular that is supposed to happen. You might initially become frustrated when you notice the inner workings of the mind that are usually on autopilot, but see if you can have a playful curiosity in discovering your own mind's nature, knowing that it will change with time and practice. Even the masters' minds still wander in meditation; they simply ignore it and maintain meditative focus.

CONCENTRATION: WITNESSING THE SENSES

The limb of *pratyahara* teaches us to call the senses away from the outer world, back to their inner source. To the beginner, this means quieting the sensory input. Intermediate practice is about exploring the nature and function of each sense organ. Advanced practice has the senses attuned to the subtlety of spirit. As one steadies *manomaya kosha*, there is a higher level of mindfulness—a greater attunement to the inner workings of the mind and body.

This exercise gives you a chance to experiment with what is usually an automatic process: hearing. You can adapt this exercise to the other senses as well, perhaps by watching a busy street, tasting or smelling something pungent, or touching something unusual. The key, as in all mindfulness practices, is to witness objectively, without judgment, so the truth of the situation can be revealed. Watch how that monkey mind creates thoughts, emotions, and stories to categorize, judge, and interpret the stimuli. Remember that the stimulus is neutral and the mind's projections turn it into something potentially disruptive. Eventually, this practice can be applied to the sensory experience of arthritis symptoms for greater equanimity and steadiness of mind:

1. Place yourself in a relaxed position, seated, or reclined. Pick a disruptive or annoying sound that often disturbs your peace of mind or meditation practice. This might be dogs barking, a dripping tap, phone notifications, or any other sound that repeats in intervals and bothers you.

2. Select an uplifting focus (see the Meditation Sampler in this chapter for ideas) and set your mind there. As the disruptive sound occurs and draws your attention away from the meditative focus, notice the specific thoughts that come up, then draw the mind back to its focus. There are often several thoughts before we even notice that the mind has wandered. If you practice this exercise over time, you will perceive that the mind will not wander as far when the disruption occurs; it becomes easier to get and stay focused.

3. After you have practiced acknowledging the mind's habits and returning to your focus several times, pause for contemplation. Consider the content of the thoughts that arise in response to the disruption. What might be underlying such thoughts? Is it anger that the barking dogs aren't being cared for, worry about the water bill, an addictive pull to the phone? There are likely many reasons why the disruption draws your attention. Seek as many as possible in order to better understand the workings of your mind.

4. If possible, come up with a neutral or soothing response to the mind's upset stories. "Dogs bark; it's as simple as that." "I commit to replacing the washer on the dripping tap." "Meditation increases dopamine so I don't need to check my phone so often to soothe myself. Whatever is on the other side of that notification can wait a few minutes."

5. Interact with the disruptive sound again, this time allowing it to be present without attaching the emotionally-driven story/reaction. Remind yourself

of the neutralizing point of view from Step 4, and return to your meditative focus again and again. In time, you won't notice the disruptions anymore.

When we acknowledge the mental patterns that make the disruption so strong, we gain understanding into the workings of *manomaya kosha*. It is possible to tell a different tale and not have the same emotional reactions to external stimuli. This is true even when the stimulus is joint pain. You control how much energy you give it. You write the story you tell yourself. Soon, the mind forms a new relationship with the stimuli. You understand that mind tends to work on habit and it is possible to choose thoughts and direct your focus where you want it. The number of disruptive thoughts are fewer and the neutral response soothes sooner.

BREATHING: COOLING BREATH: *SHEETALI*

When one gains greater control over the depth, rhythm, and even style of breathing, it is a stronger platform for *manomaya kosha*. The breath supports the nervous system in remaining calm and balanced, which is necessary for the mind to focus. While any breathing practice can help balance energy and steady a busy mind, the following breathing practice has the added benefit of cooling the body's systems:

1. Curl the tongue and stick it out or if that is not possible, create an "O" with the lips as if you were sipping through a straw.

2. Inhale slowly, gently, and long through the straw of the tongue or lips along the back of the tongue, through the trachea to the lungs.

3. Exhale through the nose. Allow the mind and body to relax as you focus on breathing.

4. Continue this for anywhere from 30 seconds to five minutes. Do you notice your tongue becoming cool and dry? Imagine this cool permeating the lungs, transferring to the blood, where it is carried to every cell in the body to quell the heat.

Almost any breathing practice, so long as it is healthy for you, will help calm your mind and body. In fact, if a breathing practice creates stress, it may be a clue to avoid it for a while. A yoga therapist will be able to help personalize a plan of healthy practices to ensure that the breathwork, movements, and mental practices are in alignment with clients' unique intentions and requirements. The following exercise offers readers a journey through meditation styles in order to discern the types that are the best fit for their minds, dispositions, and learning needs.

CONCENTRATION: MEDITATION SAMPLER

Concentration practices and the state of meditation balance the mental *kosha*. For reasons discussed earlier this chapter, meditation could be considered an antidote to pain. There are as many ways to meditate as there are minds to focus. If you practice a variety, you will learn which ones work best for you in various situations. You can tell the style that suits you because it will seem to come naturally and the amount of time you practice it will seem shorter. You may also revisit the relaxation, visualization, and breathing practices offered in chapters throughout this book. The more tools in the toolbox, the more likely you are to be able to address your needs in the moment, or support your clients in doing the same:

1. Find a comfortable practice space for roughly 15 minutes when you will be undisturbed. Set a timer on your phone for 2 or 3 minutes. Make sure the alarm is soothing and nonintrusive, perhaps with a gradual volume increase or nature sounds, so that you are not shocked out of your meditation session. Find a comfortable position that allows the natural sweep of the spine. If you are sitting on the floor rather than a chair, use whatever props are required to raise the pelvis and support the lower joints. You can also try standing up or reclining if that is more comfortable.

2. Activate the timer and begin to focus on the breath. Allow a natural breath; in other words, do not interfere with its movement. Relax as you focus on and trust the innate intelligence of the breath. If your mind wanders, simply bring it back to the movement of the breath. Continue this process until the timer rings.

3. Take time to notice your sense of mental clarity, physical relaxation, emotions, or anything else that arises. You may journal the effects and insights resulting from this practice.

4. Select a peaceful or happy image, such as a scene in nature, the face of a loved one, or spiritual symbol. Note, this is not a moving picture but a still image. If you are not visual, you may use another sense, such as imagining a sound, flavor, aroma, or feeling. Focus your mind's eye on this still image (or other sense impression), drawing your attention back each time it wanders. When the timer rings, repeat Step 3.

5. Select a word or short phrase and repeat it slowly in your mind. Extend the vowels and, if applicable, leave pauses between words. Perceive the meaning behind the language. Bring your mind back when it drifts. Repeat Step 3 when the timer rings.

6. Engage in a mindfulness practice, just observing any information coming in through the senses. Notice the thoughts and feelings happening within you, without judging them or trying to change them. Watch your inner world until the timer rings, then repeat Step 3.

7. Connect to something spiritually meaningful. You may pray, talk to your Higher Power, or consider the wisdom of the natural world. An especially powerful application is loving kindness, where you focus on compassion for yourself, you own body, and even the condition of arthritis. If you begin thinking rather than connecting, bring your awareness back to a sense of "something more." When the timer rings, repeat Step 3.

Some of these techniques will be more aligned with your needs than others. You may have even noticed yourself bringing your most comfortable focus into the other practices. For example, a mantra meditator attempting the visualization process of picturing a tree will wind up reciting "Tree...tree...tree..." while holding only a vague sensory impression of the tree itself.

Meditate in the ways that feel most comfortable and natural to you. Remaining faithful to meditation is challenging enough; do not challenge yourself with the technique you choose. For an investigation and theory of categories of meditations, check out Robert Butera's *Meditation for Your Life*. Let a focused mind support you as your meditation practice grows.

When Meditation Seems Impossible

There will be days that are difficult to meditate. All focus may return to the pain, whether physical, mental, or emotional. Perhaps the mind races too much to calm down or stress levels are too high. Meditating on how much pain you are in, or how hard it is to meditate, is counterproductive. It is recommended that when the mind continually refocuses on a problem, be it a physical sensation, worry or other harmful concerns—that we not attempt meditation. What we focus on during meditation becomes stronger within us; thus, some days it is better to not meditate at all. However, if may be possible to use meditation as a tool for changing your automatic reactions to pain.

Instead of focusing on how much pain you are in, see if you can observe the pain without stories about what it means, what it says about your past or future or what emotions it elicits. Don't try to ignore the pain, but also don't allow it your full attention. Notice it along with any other sensory information that surrounds you, including the taste in your mouth, the smells in the room, the sounds outside. Avoid personally attaching or identifying with the pain. The pain may linger for a long time or it may dissipate. But the pain is not you. You existed before the pain and you will exist after it. The pain is just an experience you are having, like any other experience. Some experiences are positive and some are negative. Meditation is about stepping back from the attachment to any single experience, allowing them each to come and go in time.

If you are able, you may even use the pain as an opportunity to cultivate love for the body and mental acceptance. Loving-kindness meditation, where you focus each breath on a sense of appreciation and acceptance for your whole self, can help alter your relationship with pain. The painful stimulus actually becomes a cue to remember relaxation and self-love. This is a way of building wisdom and finding genuine appreciation for yourself, your body, and even the condition of arthritis. By focussing on loving-kindness instead of lamenting the pain, it actually helps distance your sense of self and internal experience *away* from the symptoms. This de-identification with the sensory information is a form of *pratyahara*, or sense mastery, which has been discussed earlier. Similarly, by bringing the attention to loving-kindness, it changes the "story" associated with the pain. This further helps the brain develop in the direction of ease.

There are numerous options for applying yogic focus, ease, and relaxation that do not involve traditional meditation. Perform a relaxation from this book or listen to a guided meditation. Gentle movements to lubricate the joints and ease tired muscles are an excellent point of focus and can help with many symptoms. Walking meditation, where you link breath to your steps or are fully present with your body and surroundings, is a superb means of mental focus. Mindfulness, or full and active presence moment-to-moment, during routine activities is a common—not to mention efficient—form of meditation. Journaling, drawing, coloring, or talking to a trusted friend are all ways of expressing yourself authentically and with dedicated attention, but are active enough that they do not create an internal downward spiral the way meditation might on a rough day.

When it is difficult to meditate in stillness, when focus is elusive or awareness sticks on pain or harm, it is okay to apply other tools of movement, attention, relaxation, or expression instead. On such days, you might consider those activities to be your meditation practice, so long as your full presence of mind is involved. If you are a beginner, remember that meditation is challenging for everyone and your dedication matters! Meditation doesn't have to be seated. It also doesn't have to be easy. Just stick with a commitment to practice and know that you are literally changing the structure of your brain and its activity for the better, even if it doesn't seem like anything is happening.

Summary

The experience of pain is a complex one, involving numerous physiological and psychological factors. It is important to build a healthcare team you trust in order to cope. Self-care strategies that balance emotions and state of mind can change the brain's response to pain, as well as pain's impact on the brain! Yoga practices, notably meditation, benefit the body and mind of those suffering with arthritis and related conditions. These strategies directly affect one's ability to perceive and cope with pain. Yoga practices impact the CNS and brain function—even changing the size and shape of the brain. Yoga also brings many mental health benefits, which I will discuss in the next chapter.

Chapter 8

ARTHRITIS AND A
HEALTHY MIND

We continue exploring *manomaya kosha*, the mental layer, by investigating the mental health components associated with arthritis. Stress, depression, and anxiety are common for people living with arthritis, and yoga, in conjunction with professional mental health support, can help to manage these challenges. In this chapter, you will find a brief overview of stress, anxiety, and depression in arthritis and numerous practices to support you or your clients in maintaining good mental health while coping with chronic disease.

Stress and Arthritis

Stress management and self-care are crucial for people with arthritis. Daily stresses can exacerbate pain, affect psychological health, and contribute to disability.[107] In fact, higher levels of pain are reported on days of greater stress.[108] Therapies that focus on stress reduction show decreased pain, supporting the connection between stress and arthritis symptoms.[109]

Many people living with arthritis know that psychological stress can have an impact on arthritis symptoms. It is important to distinguish here between *stress*, which is a response, and *stressor*, which is the incident associated with that response. The way a person perceives a situation, and how stressful it may be, is impacted by a variety of personal factors. These include genetics, coping strategies, personal history, and other life circumstances. One individual situation, like a challenging co-worker, might not seem overwhelming by itself, but taken in context with other life challenges, including all that is required to manage arthritis, it can feel much more overwhelming.

The perception of stress, whether it is a result of one major stressor or several minor ones, impacts the body's physiology. Our body is designed to respond appropriately to threats of physical harm, like hunger or wild predators. If we encounter a bear, for example, a short-term burst of redirected blood flow and other physiological changes can help us to be more effective, and hopefully to survive. After the situation is resolved (we escape from the bear), our physiology returns to normal.

In the case of chronic stressors that don't easily resolve, these physiological response are not only useless, they can actually be harmful to our health. The compounding of this physiological overactivity is called "allostatic load" and fortunately, the practices of yoga can help to reverse the stress response and bring the body into a more balanced physiology, despite external challenges.

As I talk about elsewhere in this book, there are ways people living with arthritis can make lifestyle choices that actually change the stressors in their lives. I have known people to end relationships, change jobs, and otherwise reduce their obligations. Such drastic measures are not always possible, however, and this brings to mind the philosophy behind the Serenity Prayer, which has been foundational in the addiction recovery movement: "God, grant me the serenity to accept the things I cannot change, the courage to change the things I can, and the wisdom to know the difference." While this need not necessarily be considered a prayer to God, the concepts in it are very relevant to managing chronic disease. In some cases, you may be able to actually change the stressor itself. In other cases, the circumstance can't be changed, but your perspective about the circumstance can change. I think of this as actually going beyond acceptance to reframe the situation and therefore the way your body and brain are affected by it.

The stress that impacts arthritis is the *stress response*, not the *stressor*, and this is affected by our perceptions and perspective. For example, do you see the situation as a threat, a challenge, or an opportunity? Is it an obstacle or an adventure in self-discovery? Does it overwhelm or demonstrate your resilience? These changes in your perception of the situation are not necessarily easy, but the philosophy and practices of yoga can help facilitate a shift in the direction of better stress management and reduced perceived stress. Even when it isn't easy to change the way you perceive a situation, the tools of yoga can certainly dampen the severity of the physiological response. By lessening the allostatic load, it is possible to reduce the impact if stress on pain and mental health.

Depression and Anxiety in People with Arthritis

While arthritis is the leading cause of disability in the US, depression is the leading cause of disability worldwide.[110] Pain, isolation, lack of energy, and limited social engagement or community support affect all aspects of a person with arthritis, including mental health. Physical limitations are a chronic source of stress,[111] and mental health issues such as depression and anxiety are commonly comorbid with arthritis (i.e. they occur together). A greater proportion of individuals with arthritis are reported to have depression compared to individuals without arthritis,[112] which is partly due to the challenges of life with arthritis, but, as discussed in Chapter 9, may also be related to the systemic inflammation associated with autoimmune arthritis.

Depression is characterized by low mood and diminished interest or pleasure in most activities. Many of its symptoms, like changes in weight, sleep, and motor control or loss of energy and concentration, also occur in arthritis. Arthritis and related conditions can be so debilitating, or create so much extra effort in daily life, that they narrow enjoyment until there is very little left in the average day. People with arthritis become depressed about not only the loss of their own health and changes in self-image, but also the loss of jobs, relationships, and activities that were important to them. Fatigue can be so intense that it may be difficult for a person with arthritis to discern whether they are depressed or simply battling common symptoms of arthritis.

Similarly, some symptoms of anxiety, like fatigue, trouble sleeping, or difficulty concentrating, overlap with arthritis symptoms. People with arthritis commonly report being anxious about triggering a flare with their lifestyle choices or falling and injuring themselves. Anxiety is typically a response to perceived future danger, in other words, worry. From a clinical perspective, it is worrying that is hard to control and lasts for days. Anxiety has physiological symptoms, too, as described in the section above on stress, and impairs important areas of life such as relationships, job, and personal interests.

People who are depressed or anxious experience greater levels of pain, and mood disturbances have been associated with higher levels of inflammation. Unfortunately, depression and anxiety are more common for arthritis patients than they are in the general population. One-third of people with arthritis also have a mood disorder such as depression or anxiety. The mechanisms involved in this relationship may include changes in brain activity, inflammation, pain processes, and the challenges of life with a chronic, unpredictable disease. Fortunately, there are a variety of effective methods for treating depression and anxiety, including talk therapy and medications. Some components of yoga may also improve depression and anxiety, such as physical activity, relaxation practices, and shifts in personal philosophy and perspective.

The Unexpected Relationship between Depression and Anxiety

Depression and anxiety may seem opposite but they actually relate to one another. Although they do not necessarily move in sync, where there is one you often find the other. I often think of them as two sides of the same coin. They each disrupt one's health in many ways by altering thoughts, mood, activity, sleep, and appetite. Depression may present as an absence of energy, while anxiety seems like too much nervous energy. Depression might coincide with thoughts of the past and anxiety the future; neither allows for the presence yoga brings.

Yoga philosophy teaches that everything in the material world is subject to three forces: inertia (*tamas*), overactivity (*rajas*), or balanced purity (*sattva*). These forces, or constituents of nature, are called *gunas* in Sanskrit and they can be applied to the foods we eat, our leisure activities and even our thoughts, emotions, and beliefs. Depression is an imbalance of *tamas,* where lowered mood, energy, and interest are evident. Anxiety, with the high nervous system activity, rushing thoughts, and intense emotions, is an imbalance of *rajas*. I was even part of a research team beginning to conceptualize the modern polyvagal theory as a neurophysiological counterpart to the *gunas*.[113]

While many people living with arthritis suffer from mood disorders, or imbalances in the gunas related to *manomaya kosha*, mood fluctuations are not necessarily negative. In fact, similar moods can feel positive or negative, which may be due to whether we are experiencing the mood from a place of balance or imbalance. Some examples from the Profile of Positive and Negative Mood States might include: strong/hostile, excited/jittery, or alert/afraid. The moods in each pair are similar, but with very different connotations. Some of the work of improving mood through yoga may be in shifting that balance toward more positive moods.

In our Yoga for Arthritis study at Johns Hopkins,[114] we found that yoga improved positive moods but did not reduce negative moods when comparing yoga participants to an inactive control group. This might seem counter-intuitive, but it represents a broader array of mood states. However, when we looked at all yoga participants over time, changes in both positive *and* negative moods were seen after both eight weeks of yoga and nine months later. It may be that the increase in positive mood is more robust than the decrease in negative mood. That idea might resonate with those of you who have practiced yoga.

Yoga for Arthritis studies[115] also revealed that after eight weeks of classes, students felt better able to care for themselves. They reported BPSS effects like a greater sense of calm, better focus, healthier eating habits, improved coping skills, more social connection, and pride. The yoga practice helped provide motivation and confidence to perform the self-care practices that maintain health through arthritis. Furthermore, the practices themselves were identified as coping strategies and self-care tools.

In the cases of both depression and anxiety, yoga practices like deep breathing, gentle movement, and relaxation can restore mental and emotional balance. Cardiovascular exercise is also known to be effective in helping to manage symptoms of both anxiety and depression. Unfortunately, when feeling depressed, it can be hard to muster the motivation to take action; when feeling anxious, the idea of taking time for self-care can seem elusive. If you, a client or a loved one is feeling symptoms of depression and anxiety that are unyielding, seek the guidance of a qualified professional. Both talk therapy and medication are available in many forms and enhance the effects of self-care practices like deep breathing and exercise. Similarly, someone who is using medication for mood management might consider the addition of talk therapy and/or self-care practices for greater efficacy.

Just as some forms of arthritis require medication to help manage a dysregulated immune system, the same is true for some mood disorders. Mental health conditions are often ignored and untreated, which is partly due to cultural stigma. While self-care practices may help to reduce medication dose or severity, there are many factors that impact disease states and judgment regarding whether medication is appropriate should be left to the individual and their team of care providers. The consequences of not getting help when it is needed are too great for anyone to feel judged about doing so.

REFLECTION: *GUNAS* REFLECTION EXERCISE

The *gunas*, or constituents of manifested reality, are at play in our everyday lifestyle. The qualities of inertia, agitation, and balance show up in our thoughts, behaviors, relationships, sleep habits, and even the entertainment we choose and foods we eat. The relationship between lifestyle and *gunas* is bi-directional. What we put into our minds and bodies, through thought or action, we get out in feeling and belief. Similarly, our beliefs and feelings influence what we choose to take in. The following exercise gives you a chance to understand the connection between the energies you are engaging in your life and how you are thinking and feeling. You may also review these questions with clients to help improve awareness about healthy lifestyle choices.

REFLECTION QUESTION #1: EMOTIONAL RESPONSES

What are your prevalent emotions through the day? When something doesn't go your way, how do you tend to feel about it? How long does that feeling last? What is it like for you when you are happy or looking forward to something? How long does that last? In general, are your feelings low, high, or balanced? In what ways do you keep your emotions calm?

REFLECTION QUESTION #2: NUTRITIONAL HABITS

What is your favorite meal? For what reasons? When you need a snack, what do you tend to choose? What kinds of foods do you you tend to crave (sweets, spicy, heavy, creamy, etc.)? What do you tell yourself to make it okay to eat these things? How do you feel after you succumb to cravings? How does that food digest, considering a few hours later as well as the next day or two? What, if any, are your strategies for planning, preparing, and eating meals rich in vegetables, lean proteins, and healthy fats? How do you feel after you eat healthful meals? How do they digest (over hours and days)?

REFLECTION QUESTION #3: FREE TIME

When you don't have to be anywhere or do anything, how do you choose to spend your time? When you are busy, what do you long to be doing instead? What do you spend a lot of time doing that you would rather do less of? What activity do you think is going to help you feel better but actually doesn't? When you are rested and feeling well, what activities do you enjoy?

REFLECTION QUESTION #4: RELATIONSHIPS

Who do you spend the most time with? Who would you *choose* to spend the most time with? Who supports you? Who loves you unconditionally? When you are with your friends, what tends to be the content of your conversation (current events, gossip, philosophy, science, jokes, personal growth, sports, etc.)? In what specific ways do your relationships nourish you? How do you contribute to and maintain meaningful connections?

REFLECTION QUESTION #5: THE FUTURE

When you imagine your "Future Self," what images, ideas, and hopes come to mind? What goals are you working towards? What choices are you making to protect your future (health, finances, emotional wellbeing, etc.)? Are there secret wishes you carry?

Now, go back through those reflections questions and note the ones that are dominant in *tamas* (low emotions, junk foods, shallow relationships, etc.), *rajas* (hyper/agitated, competitive, stimulated, overworked, tense, etc.), or *sattva* (peaceful, cooperative/contributing, meaningful/purposeful, equanimous, relaxed, healthy, enriching, etc.). People with depression are likely *tamasic* in other areas as well. Similarly, those with anxiety are likely dominated by *rajas*.

Select one habit you can shift in the direction of *sattva* and plan simple strategies to implement that change. In what aspect of life are you most interested in creating balance? Remember, it's important to approach the movement to *sattva* with a *sattvic* (balanced, peaceful) approach! A richer emotional life is possible through awareness and conscious lifestyle choices. This is what makes consistent effort (*tapas*) so important in alleviating mental health issues.

REFLECTION: SELF-CARE THROUGH ESTABLISHED PRACTICE

Some kind of daily self-care practice is essential for inner peace. One of the first limbs of yoga (*niyama*) emphasizes the importance of consistent effort. This can be journaling, going for a walk, or eating lots of veggies and legumes. It can also be a daily yoga practice. When you feel empowered to practice yoga on your own, you get to enjoy yoga's benefits whenever you want! This book is written so that you can dive in to safe, simple practices that benefit your wellbeing physically, energetically, emotionally, mentally, and spiritually:

1. Without thinking too much, take 30 seconds and jot down as many reasons as possible why you want to practice yoga. It's okay if you repeat yourself—that can help the flow of ideas.

2. Circle the motivators that are most important to you. Take a few deep breaths as you imagine and feel those reasons filling, calming, and healing you.

3. Think of your average day. When are there 5–15 minute pockets of time where you could insert simple movements, meditations, or breathing practices? It is best to think of these times as segments of your day (first thing in the morning, after work, before dinner, etc.) rather than specific times on the clock. Record your answers, possibly by setting a reminder on your phone. This isn't to tell yourself to actually practice at those times; instead, it cues you to notice that you have the option during those segments of your day.

4. If you were to practice, what types of practice interest and inspire you most? You may skim through this or other yoga books for ideas. I have been careful to include practices for arthritis symptoms in each chapter. Briefly list these most compelling practices, perhaps marking the page or writing down the page number, so you have them as a future reminder.

5. Pick one time of day and one practice to commit to. No amount of practice is wasted, so it's fine to start with just a few minutes. Every effort towards better mental and physical health is worthy and has benefit. Furthermore, time spent on self-care fills the space that might otherwise be taken up

by harmful behaviors like addictions or despair. Write down the specific practice(s) you will employ and where in your schedule you will fit them.

6. Do it! You don't have to begin with daily efforts; even twice per week will facilitate improvement over time, often in unexpected and uplifting ways. In no time, you will *want* to practice every day!

This exploration into your motivation, convenience, and interest sets you up for success and greater mental health as you gently and systematically bring yoga into your daily life. Remember that a few minutes each day can lead to powerful shifts in life on all levels. Start small, be consistent, and accept yourself as the process unfolds.

RELAXATION: AWARENESS RELAXATION

The following relaxation takes you on a journey through the *koshas*, sequentially relaxing each layer of your being, or that of a patient or client you may be sharing it with. This practice is often used in our Yoga for Arthritis trainings and classes. It is suitable for beginners and can be performed during times of mental and physical pain, stress, or flares:

1. *Prepare*: Lie on your back for deep relaxation. If you would like, you can prop yourself up or cover yourself over with blankets to be more comfortable. Take a few deep breaths to release into this reclined position. It is okay to use another position of you cannot get comfortable lying on your back.

2. *Tense and Release*: We will tense and release the body three times, lifting arms, legs, and head an inch above the floor and squeezing every muscle in the body. 1, 2, 3…squeeze tighter and tighter, then release and drop into the floor. 1, 2, 3…lift again and use every muscle from head to toe, then release and let go. Last time, 1, 2, 3…tighten every muscle and use up all of your energy so there is nothing left to do but relax.

3. Let it all go: Make any adjustments so that you can be comfortable, balanced, and still for the next few minutes. Notice every point of connection that

the body makes with the floor and deepen those points of connection by dropping and releasing to the pull of gravity.

4. *Body Scan*: Become aware of the tips of your toes. Allow all of the muscles in the toes to relax. Feel that sense of relaxation in the toes start to move up through the body to the balls of the feet, arches, heels, tops of the feet, and ankles. Let the relaxation move up to the lower legs, knees, thighs, and hips. Feel the sacrum sinking into the floor and the pelvis widen. Allow the abdominal muscles and organs to sink in toward the lower back. From the waist down, you are completely relaxed.

5. Become aware of your fingertips: Feel the muscles of the fingers letting go and let that relaxation move up to the knuckles, hands, and wrists. Let it travel into the forearms, elbows, upper arms, and shoulders. The arms and legs are totally relaxed.

6. Become aware of your center: Soften everything around the navel and feel that relaxation moving up the sides of the torso and the spine into the ribcage, chest, and upper back, all around the shoulder blades and collarbones. Everything from the neck down is fully relaxed.

7. Notice the heart and the sense of warmth and light coming from the heart, moving out through the whole body and into the space around you. Let that sense of calm travel up and relax the neck and throat, jaw, and tongue. All of the muscles of the face and head let go and surrender to relaxation. The whole body is now relaxed.

8. *Breath Awareness*: Become aware of your breath. Notice the breath rise and fall, flowing in and out of the body like a wave. Follow the breath as it becomes slower, deeper, and softer, allowing the body to relax even more with every exhale. Trust the breath to bring in what the body needs and let go of what it doesn't need.

9. *Mental/Intellectual Awareness*: Notice any thoughts that might be moving through the mind. Let the thoughts fade. Release any thoughts that aren't serving you. Tuck away the ones you want to keep for another time. Allow the mind to be clear and open, relaxed along with the breath and body. Spend a few moments enjoying this time with no expectations or demands, just be here in this moment, with a natural sense of inner peace.

10. *Return to Seated*: Become aware of the breath again. Allow it to deepen, bringing energy back into the body and out to the fingers and toes. Allow the fingers and toes to wiggle. The head might rock side to side. You can reach, stretch, twist, or move in whatever way feels right, bringing yourself onto one side in the fetal position for a few more breaths. Gently bring yourself back up to a seated position.

11. *Spiritual Centering*: Sit up tall with the shoulders back and down, long spine, relaxed body, deep breath, and clear mind. You may choose to close with a chant or prayer that is meaningful to you. Perhaps just think of a word that holds meaning and repeat aloud or in your mind.

After three repetitions, allow yourself to rest in silence. Notice a sense of inner tranquility and peacefulness all around you. You might want to hold your focus on the breath, an image, or an intention. When you notice your mind wandering away from that focus, bring it back with acceptance and understanding, knowing that this will become easier with time and practice.

This systematic relaxation and focus on peaceful inner qualities helps foster greater ease in body and mind. Aspects of this practice can be used anytime, anywhere, as the body is systematically relaxed, stressful thoughts released, and the mind focused on a sense of peace. Your personal chant, prayer, or intention can be repeated throughout the day to help cultivate a sense of inner peace in the face of anxiety or depression.

BREATHING: BALANCING WITH *NADI SODHANA* BREATH

A common breathing practice to balance emotions and stress response is alternate nostril breathing, or *nadi sodhana*. The *nadis* are the meridians that the *prana* travels through and *sodhana* means "cleansing" or "balance." This practice can help you or your clients shift from a state of *rajas* or *tamas* to one of balance and equanimity (*sattva*). One study measured the effects of this practice on heart rate variability and inhale/exhale ratios and found that alternate nostril breathing is beneficial in increasing parasympathetic (relaxed) tone. Healthcare practitioners may share this balancing practice with patients. What is provided here is a beginner's version. Some approaches to this practice include pauses after the inhale/exhale and varying breath counts. If at any time you feel dizzy or like you are not getting enough air, simply stop and breathe normally:

1. Close your right nostril with your right index finger and exhale through the left nostril. Now inhale through the left nostril for approximately six beats.

2. Seal your left nostril with left index finger, release right nostril, and exhale through the right side for approximately six beats. Inhale through the right nostril. You have now completed a full round of *nadi sodhana*.

3. Seal right nostril, release left nostril, and exhale. Notice this is the same as Step 1. Continue repeating the above steps for ten rounds of breath. When you have completed the practice, take time to notice its impact on your energy, thoughts, emotions, relaxation, and other effects throughout your whole system.

Nadi sodhana is a balancing and cleansing practice. It works on the three main channels in PMK to support health, ease, and wisdom. This practice calls forth equilibrium and calm while supporting the body in adapting to stress more readily, thereby helping to regulate emotions. Apply this practice to soothe overwhelm and frustration, animating you when depressed and soothing you when anxious.

CONCENTRATION: *PRATYAHARA:* CALLING THE SENSES INWARD

We live in an overstimulated culture. Our sense organs are bombarded throughout the day with flashing screens, billboards, traffic sounds, media noise, and more. This level of stimulation makes it challenging for the emotions, mind, and nervous system to relax, which can exacerbate mental health issues like depression and anxiety. Even when we seek quiet spaces, the impressions of the world around us continue to impose themselves upon the mind, which makes it difficult to attune to our own inner wisdom and peace. The following practice helps you regain a more balanced mental state by focusing the senses inwards:

1. Sit outside or near a window. Look around you then close your eyes and simply notice what your mind does. What do you think about? How does it

make you feel? What images, sounds, memories or chatter show up? How believable is each thought?

2. Now gaze at one aspect of nature, such as the sky, a tree, or flowers. If you cannot see any nature, gaze at a nearby picture or object. Allow your eyes to relax as they take in the input. Become passive as you look. Do not "try" to see anything; rather, allow the eyes to receive the image. Feel the eyes, brow, and jaw relaxing. It's okay if the eyes unfocus, just allow them to rest on your chosen object and receive the visual information. If your mind wanders, bring it back to relaxing your eyes, forehead, and breath. You may even imagine relaxing the optic nerve and brain as you lightly gaze.

3. Close the eyes and perceive the darkness on the back of your eyelids. Notice the sounds that your ears receive, without attempting to hear anything. Just as your eyes became passive in the previous step, allow the ears to rest. Keep the breath, face, and jaw relaxed.

4. Notice the difference in the speed, content, and quality of your thoughts. What emotions are with you? Is your internal world quieter, calmer, or more settled?

5. When you return to the world, do so slowly and with awareness. You may notice that your senses are more keen or sensitive.

The ability to rein in the senses and be comfortable with silence support peace of mind. When the sensory environment is quieter, it requires fewer resources to focus on what is important; thus, it is less energetically, emotionally, and mentally tiring. Practice this exercise anytime you feel fatigued or overstimulated in order to balance yourself.

REFLECTION: REMOVING OBSTACLES TO PRACTICE

There are often barriers to caring for ourselves. Busyness, time limits, fatigue, pain, family obligations, and unhealthy habits are just a few of the obstacles to employing yoga practice. Remember, "yoga" doesn't just mean postures. Anything you perform mindfully could fit under this umbrella: music, sport, relaxation, preparing meals, etc. Follow this system, based on the ethics of truthfulness (*satya*) and effort (*tapas*), to help yourself or clients continue a steady daily practice:

1. If you have not already gone through the process earlier in this chapter, Self-Care through Established Practice, begin there. Those steps set you up for initial success. It can be challenging, however, to maintain a practice—no matter how motivated one is.

2. Thinking back to the last few times you missed your yoga/meditation practice (or other meaningful daily practice like journaling, walking, connecting with loved ones, etc.), jot down what got in your way. Was it symptoms from the arthritis, thoughts you were having, things you would rather have been doing…?

3. Call upon the part of yourself that is interested in yoga, misses it or is connected to the range of benefits it brings. For each of the reasons in step 2, provide a motivating response. For example, "Even though my pain and fatigue were terrible, I would like to lay in bed and feel my diaphragm rise and fall," "Thoughts that the yoga doesn't help or that I'm too tired to do anything go away when I recite my affirmation. I feel better mentally and physically!" or "Even though I would rather be doing the dishes while I have the energy, or watching TV after a rough day, just a few movements lower my pain levels over time…and when I miss my yoga, the pain gets worse over time" or "You can do it!" Personalize the responses and tell yourself the truth.

4. Ask yourself if there are other ways you can unwind these obstacles, such as practicing during a different segment of your day, incorporating more fun or creativity or acknowledging the immediate effects of each practice you apply. Keeping a journal of your yoga practice is an excellent way to track the benefits. It is human to forget what things were like before we began yoga practice, how much we struggle at first or some of the insights that arise from practice. The journal offers reminders and inspiration.

5. Keep these responses handy. The next time you are tempted to disregard practice altogether, read through this list and offer yourself one small aspect of yoga. This can be a single deep breath, a moment to gaze at nature, or, like Terri in this chapter, a single, meaningful posture.

Small, simple efforts towards a steady practice can make a huge difference in quality of life, especially over long periods of time. Be truthful with yourself about why you want to practice and continue with small, consistent steps. For more support in developing a home practice and staying consistent with yoga, seek one of the hundreds of Yoga for Arthritis teachers whom I have trained internationally. If there is not one in your area, check the resources in this book on how to find the right teacher for you.

POSTURE: TERRI'S STRONG MOUNTAIN

One of my many inspiring students, Terri, offers a great example for the use of metaphor in *asana* and for mental health. It is stated continually throughout this book that it is not the form of the posture that is important, as much as the attitude or archetype of its essence. When we align with these ancient states and symbols, we alter our perspectives, physiology, and psychology. Terri, a student who now has multiple arthritis diagnoses, embodied this approach.

Due to unbearable family circumstances, Terri was missing yoga class, flying back and forth between her home in Maryland and her family in Florida. It was understandable that with everything she was going through, she could not attend regularly. She did not have the time or energy for a full home practice but she knew it was important to her wellbeing and wanted to find a way to keep her practice alive. When she returned, I asked her if she had been practicing at all. She told me that the only pose she used during this trying time was Mountain. She wanted to see if this yoga stuff really worked, and she knew that she needed to *be* a mountain. She created a game with her grandchildren, in which they all pretended to be mountains. She even stood in Mountain while doing the dishes. She reported that this simple practice helped her get through a difficult time. Terri says that these many years later, she still practices Mountain pose in the pool as her challenge of the day. Since learning yoga, she also now knows that if she feels achy, she can get down on the floor and stretch. Remaining limber has helped her to stay active as she ages.

To many yoga students, Mountain Pose is just a fancy way of saying "stand still." However, when one incorporates the attitude and archetype of the pose, there is a deep connection to steadiness, balance, fortitude, greatness, provision, expansiveness, and many other qualities one may attribute to mountains. Terri practiced Mountain Pose and, *being* the mountain, in posture and attitude, got her through.

Try it for yourself! Bring your feet hip-width apart (the width of the hip joints, not the flesh). Legs are strong with the knees unlocked, pelvis in neutral with a lifted but relaxed floor, the spine sweeping tall with its natural curves. Shoulders are stable, relaxed back and down without tension or slouching. Arms hang loosely at the sides. Jaw is unclenched. Gaze is soft and straight ahead.

Bring awareness to the soles of your feet. Soften the feet into the floor. Imagine that you are a part of the bedrock, deep in the earth, rising through the soil and growing into the clouds. The legs are strong and ancient stone, supporting your tall, relaxed back and the summit across the shoulders. Imagine your head as the peak of the mountain—the upper limits communing with the sun and sky. You may imagine all the kinds of life that you support as a mountain: grasses and herbs, trees and streams, birds and climbing wildlife. You are strong and balanced, capable and present. You don't have to take action of any kind. You have the right to "just BE"; this is true because you exist. Any time you feel frail, overwhelmed, or unimportant, shape yourself into a mountain and bask in that strong, sturdy presence.

Summary

Mental health concerns go hand in hand with arthritis symptoms. Yoga philosophy and practices can support better mental health through increased self-care, decreased symptoms, and improved mental outlook. Yoga can change the way one relates to arthritis, in thought, belief, self-perception, and behavior. The personal reflection, breathing, sense mastery, and posture practices in this chapter offer a starting point for improving mental health for people living with arthritis. The next chapter builds upon this by seeking a deeper wisdom within.

Chapter 9

WISDOM AND PERSPECTIVES ON ARTHRITIS (VIJANAMAYA KOSHA)

In the PMK model, there is a difference between the mind, *manomaya kosha*, the realm of thoughts and feelings, and the intellect, *vijnanamaya kosha*, the realm of realized knowledge, beliefs and wisdom. While the mind is subject to fast-changing external influences, the intellect is established and does not change much throughout the course of a lifetime. In this chapter, we explore the importance of awareness. People living with arthritis can apply deeper intellect and the wisdom of yoga to the experience of arthritis and life itself.

The Important Role of Neutral Observation

Awareness is necessary to alter the state of mind. It is the nature of the mind to jump quickly between thoughts and feelings, which has to be observed in order for it to be altered. The wisdom layer serves as that witness, empowering us to then choose our thoughts, feelings, and responses (both internally, through perspective, and externally, through behavior). In Chapter 7, you had the opportunity to witness how your senses interplayed with your inner and outer world. As we move through the *koshas,* we go from witnessing the grosser messages of the body (pain, stiffness), to more subtle changes in energy, and then to observing emotions and responses to circumstance, and finally to the underlying thoughts and beliefs that guide our experience and everyday choices. Consistently witnessing internal experiences—the how and why of what you think—allows for the experience of greater wisdom.

Yoga teaches that all things are neutral. It is human to judge and categorize; however, the wiser we become, the broader our perspective, and the greater the ability to accept things as they are. Over time, true yoga practice provides direct experience of a calm, peacefulness that is not as available in a busy life. Simply witnessing the movement of sensation, emotion, and thought trains us to be less reactive, judgmental, or attached. We learn to approach it all with equanimity instead of feeling compelled to immediately change what is. Whatever we discover within ourselves simply is at that time—thoughts, feelings, beliefs, fears, etc. It does not serve us to judge or deny these things, as they will inevitably change. And through awareness, we can help direct those changes without clinging to a need for things to be a certain way.

Anyone living with arthritis knows that change is constant. Whatever was helpful or useful may eventually stop working, whether temporarily or permanently. Arthritis symptoms may resolve and they may recur. Yoga practice teaches us to avoid feeling attached to either the challenges or the improvements. We suffer when we cling to happy things and want them to stay the same. We also suffer when we forget that pain will pass. The following exercise helps specifically develop the skill of neutral observation and non-attachment.

CONCENTRATION EXERCISE: DISCERNING THE MIND AND INTELLECT

Consider that there are (at least) two parts of your thinking self: the busy part and the calm part. You can identify these as *manomaya kosha* and *vijnanamaya kosha*, or mind and intellect/wisdom. The practice below can give you or your clients a chance to notice this distinction. While there is a part of us that feels things deeply and may be struggling, there is also a part that is already at peace, no matter the external circumstances:

1. Find a location where you will not be disturbed and find a comfortable position, sitting, standing, or reclining as needed. Do your best to keep the spine long, allowing for its natural curve. Relax the shoulders and jaw; feel the support of the floor or other surface beneath you. Allow the breath to deepen.

2. Close your eyes in order to focus inward and notice the words and images in your mind. If you aren't accustomed to this practice, it may feel strange, like you are thinking about thinking. Whatever thoughts arise in the mind; all you have to do is notice them. Soon enough, the mind will jump on to a new thought.

3. Thoughts trick us into thinking that they are interesting. When you notice you've been swept into a thought, like your grocery list, favorite movie, or that thing someone said to you, simply acknowledge the thoughts that are present and return to witnessing them.

4. After a few minutes of witnessing the thoughts and feelings—and bringing yourself back to awareness when you become absorbed in the thoughts—acknowledge that there is a part of you doing the witnessing. This wise part of you can watch without being swept up. It does not need to judge or offer commentary on the thoughts. The mind is complex and you may notice many layers within you, such as a worried layer, a caretaker layer, a what-is-this-exercise-for layer, and so on. The more you practice witnessing, the more you will connect to that inner neutrality. This wise, objective layer simply sees what is happening. It does not need to change it.

5. Jot down your observations.

6. Repeat this practice at least once per week for a few weeks. If you do, something interesting is likely to happen! You may notice that your responses to your thoughts and feelings become less attached and judgmental. By watching the thoughts and connecting to neutrality, you become more aware of, and have greater access to, the wisdom *kosha*.

The benefit of discerning between mind and wisdom is that you forge a relationship with a neutral, peaceful part of yourself. Over time, you can call upon it more readily. While this does not always help resolve a pain, it does bring comfort in remembering that there is another layer of reality. Despite everything else that may be happening or hurting, peace still resides somewhere within. Try to notice your level of neutral acceptance gradually increasing over time.

Perspectives Across a Lifetime

As one cultivates a relationship with the peaceful wisdom layer, it becomes easier to take life as it comes. Even though symptoms of arthritis may disrupt physical comfort, energy, emotions, career, activity, and relationships, there remains a calm "okay-ness" beneath the surface.

There is a difference in how people tend to cope with arthritis, depending upon their age. Anyone recently diagnosed tends to react with some aversion or denial that hopefully gradually moves towards acceptance. Because older adults have arthritis at higher rates, a diagnosis in older age may elicit less denial. Especially in the case of OA, people in their later years have an inkling that they may be developing arthritis as their joints become achy, tender, and swollen.

Those diagnosed in middle age also tend to accept the diagnosis more quickly and find ways to care for themselves and cope with the disease. Although they may resist the idea more at first, they also have the wisdom of some years to understand that arthritis and other physical ailments are a part of life.

In time, can you guess which population is the *most likely* to accept arthritis as a part of life? Acceptance is especially evident in those diagnosed when they are *young*. They seem to arrive at a certain wisdom beyond their years. Their perspectives on life, pain, suffering, challenges, and the body often wind up echoing the beliefs of people near the end of life. People diagnosed young are in a position to grapple with big questions at a tender age. Marina, introduced in Chapter 2, let go of assumptions about what her body should be able to do before she reached limits of aging. She moved into her adult years with a wise belief that her body will show up to her differently over time, rather than expecting it to remain the same. She learned at a young age that the body changes and that she must forge an active and conscious relationship with her body.

Arthritis teaches young people the wisdom of measuring expectations. Pain can be a great teacher as it guides us to shift from expectations to acceptance. It is worthy to attempt what is important, yet to also accept reality as it presents itself.

Adversity such as arthritis has the power to shift the relationship to one's own body and mind. While many regard that shift as negative, there also resides within it the seed of powerful transformation and the peace that comes with acceptance.

Approximately 300,000 children in the United States are living with arthritis. I have had the honor of working with such children, from toddlers to teens and everything in between. From my own experience, they generally seem to have greater access to their own inner wisdom than many adults. I have also worked with several young adults who were diagnosed with arthritis as children. In fact, one such individual, a burgeoning researcher, contacted me several years ago seeking employment. Jennifer Daks helped to expand Yoga for Arthritis as an organization. We also learned a lot from each other in the process. She was diagnosed with arthritis at just two and a half years old. She shares her story with you below.

Jenn's Story of Awareness and Acceptance

I began practicing yoga as part of a holistic approach to my healing journey from Juvenile Rheumatoid Arthritis (JRA). Having lived with this condition since I was a toddler, I have grown to understand the sensitivity and connection between the mind, body, and spirit. From a young age, I remember having a heightened attunement to the sensitivity of my body. At 18 months, I began limping and had swelling in my knees that became so severe I eventually couldn't even stand up on my own. Several visits to my pediatrician left me without any diagnosis. Although my doctor suspected arthritis, the test results all turned up negative. My mother recalls "pleading" with my pediatrician due to me "not getting any better." Eventually she was guided to a rheumatologist, who was the first doctor to perform an ANA test (used to diagnose autoimmune diseases such as lupus and RA) which came back positive. This test, coupled with my swelling and stiffness, led to my first diagnosis of JRA, six months after the onset of symptoms.

I was considered one of "the lucky ones" because my JRA was discovered early. After my diagnosis, I was immediately put on a DMARD (Disease-Modifying Anti-Rheumatic Drug, a type of drug used in combating RA) which, over time, reduced my swelling. Over the next few years, my symptoms gradually subsided, and at the age of seven, I officially went into a remission that lasted 11 whole years!

Growing up, I often *forgot* about my JRA. I tried many sports and grew particularly fond of gymnastics and cheerleading. Although my rheumatologist often cautioned about the high impact these sports put on my joints, I explained my love for these activities and that staying active was one of my main healing modalities. Over the years, I internalized a mantra that I would *"never"* be held back by my JRA, which seemed to be a relatively easy task for the years in remission (beyond the occasional rainy day and achy joint).

At the age of 18, I experienced my next flare up. A period of transition—moving away to college—coupled with some other stressors sent my body into *high gear.* I remember my body felt just a little stiffer each day. It didn't have the same flexibility I was used to, and my energy levels dropped. I initially assumed this was general stiffness from being less active (having recently quit cheerleading), but I knew something was seriously wrong when one morning I was unable to get out of bed on my own due to severe knee swelling. My hands were so swollen that I couldn't open the refrigerator door or even a bottle cap. I felt completely hopeless and angry at the state of my mind and body. I felt distant from my friends, as my body and energy levels seemed to be very different from others my age. I constantly viewed myself as a teenager stuck in the body of an elderly person. These thoughts felt all-encompassing—there was no break.

After 11 years of sometimes forgetting I even had JRA, my frustrations grew and I refused to welcome this experience with open arms. I was angry, resentful, sad, and confused. As my symptoms persisted despite medical interventions, I felt the need to look beyond these treatments for anything else I could do that might help. I asked my doctor what else was available and she suggested I try yoga to complement my treatment. This is when my discovery of yoga's healing powers began; I just did not consciously know it at the time.

My story isn't the flowery experience that many have when they discover yoga, but it has been a beautiful journey. The first yoga class I took was at a local gym. I distinctly remember attempting to *force* myself into a child's pose and completely hating it because my knees wouldn't bend deeply. I was in pain, grinding my teeth through the entire class. I was too nervous to ask my teacher for a modification and too upset at myself and my body for it not "doing what I wanted."

For another three years, I continued to take yoga classes sporadically, mostly hot, *vinyasa* classes. I thought: 1) This must be the only type of yoga there is, as this was the only studio in my area, and I had not taken the time to research yoga much deeper, and 2) I *should* be able to do this kind of yoga and *should* enjoy this.

Looking back, I don't think I ever completely enjoyed hot yoga. I believe what I was seeking at the time was a *solution* to my problems. I was still living by my mantra to *never* let my arthritis hold me back, so I continued, even though I could not physically keep up with the pace of class. I constantly felt as though I was one breath away from passing out every time I completed a *vinyasa*. I felt stuck in my practice, frustrated by a body that could not do the vigorous workout I had been used to. I had some internal drive to push and mold myself into this idealistic version of myself—the version of myself I had gotten used to for the past 11 years—myself in remission. Writing this now, I am realizing how heavily I relied on yoga as a physical practice and let the philosophical, spiritual, mental, and emotional components fall to the wayside. I had just begun to skim the surface of yoga.

Another year went by and I broadened my horizons to discover *hatha* yoga. I was completing a senior thesis project at this time, in which I developed a brief mindfulness-based program to relieve chronic pain and pain-related psychological symptoms in older adults. Although I could not feel it or completely believe it for myself, all of the literature I read and my instincts led me to believe in the healing power of mindfulness and yoga. I wanted to share this with others. For my project, I employed a yoga teacher to offer gentle yoga for chronic pain. In our interactions, I shared my journey with this teacher (living with arthritis and my trials with hot yoga). Having completed the Yoga for Arthritis teacher training herself, she guided me towards *hatha* yoga. She even suggested I look into the Yoga for Arthritis program to become a teacher myself (talk about setting the stage, huh?). At this point in my life, I wasn't ready to become a teacher, nor did I feel I had a strong enough practice of my own yet. I filed her advice in the back of my mind and took the first step towards focusing on a gentler and slower-paced practice.

During my first *hatha* class, I thought the gods had descended into my class and lifted me back to Heaven! I was astonished that there were actually classes out there that encouraged me to find slow, gentle release of my body that did not involve me weaving into a sweaty yoga pretzel! I began to build confidence in my practice and in myself. I began to ask my teachers for modifications and suddenly my entire practice and outlook on life began to shift. I realized, *so what* if I need to sit up on two blocks in a squat rather than the traditional look of the pose? I began to understand that the *intention* of my practice and the attitudes, beliefs, and thoughts I held could transform my life much more than just the *look* of things would. I began to become more mindful in my daily life—learning to accept pain and sensitivity as a great teacher of mine, rather than a bundle of darkness I once wanted to shove into a corner and never acknowledge. I eventually went back into remission, however I was left with idiopathic widespread chronic pain. Although it wasn't my JRA, I knew this deserved and needed the same cultivation of sensitivity and attention that JRA had called for in the past.

One of the most powerful and prominent moments in my practice thus far occurred during a yoga class one year ago. I was experiencing a lot of pain and when I arrived on my mat, I knew I would have to tailor my practice to fit my body's needs. I was moving through my *asana* into a child's pose and once again, my knees were reacting. I was unable to attain the "full expression" of this pose. Suddenly, a wave of emotions rushed over me. I could see myself in that first yoga class, struggling through my practice. Even writing this brings up those same emotions as I was, and still am, able to see my body in a similar state—with swollen joints that restrict my movement. Even though some of these restrictions still persist in my practice to this day, I am able to see the transformation of my mind, my spirit, and my body through my yogic journey. I spent the next few minutes with my head down, crying at the beautiful transformation I was seeing and experiencing in this moment. I felt completely connected; wanting to almost celebrate the pain I was feeling, welcoming it as a necessary part of myself at that moment.

Since then, I have seen my journey project in directions I had never even imagined, and I became dedicated to the study and practice of yoga. I embarked on a yoga teacher training, joined the Yoga for Arthritis team, and have dedicated my doctoral studies to investigate how yoga and mindfulness practices can help improve the lives and relationships of people living with chronic pain conditions! My experiences have taught me to embrace this journey, and learn from the obstacles, twists, and turns life may throw at us. I have learned that arthritis is much more than just a physical condition; it can impact every ounce of our being and those around us. These experiences have helped me lean into the experience of living with arthritis, pave new paths, and reinforce my commitment to empowering and supporting others to live fully with arthritis.

I hope to use all of these experiences to help others discover yoga as a gateway to gain awareness, compassion, and acceptance for themselves and the world around them. We all have limitless potential—we just need to discover what that unique trajectory looks like for each and every one of us.

POSTURE: SUBTLE *ASANA* PRACTICE

The more we practice attuning to subtle cues within us, the deeper our mindfulness capabilities become. The following attunement practice slows down a yoga posture so that it is easier to notice thoughts and sensations and make necessary adjustments. Above all else, be honest with yourself and practice accepting the requests of your body:

1. Lie down on your back in a comfortable position. Take a few three-part, conscious breaths, and check with the sensations throughout your body. Where is there comfort and discomfort? Are there areas you can relax any further? Notice the fullness and ease of each breath. If the breath is not full and easy, notice that, too. Acknowledge the thoughts and feelings that are with you. You may even notice the part of you doing the acknowledging.

2. Perform a few gentle movements. You may take inspiration from this book, a video, your personal yoga practice, or other gentle movements that are familiar or comfortable to you. Remain aware of your body, breath, thoughts, and feelings. Acknowledge if anything feels uncomfortable, if you are forcing any movements, or if your mind or breath becomes erratic.

3. Select a posture or movement that challenges or awakens you. Do not select anything that causes pain or puts you at risk. Perform it slowly and carefully, noticing the cues from your whole body, your ability to keep the breath smooth and the thoughts and feelings that arise. Respect what you witness. It is likely you will hear yourself tell a story about the discomfort, your body, the disease, etc. Do not ignore the sensation, and bring your attention back to breath as you might do in meditation. Instead, keep the breath even, continue witnessing and alter your movement or body position as needed. Aim to maintain neutrality while also responding to the sensation and disregarding the story.

4. Return to your resting position. Name what you witnessed in Step 3. You may ask yourself, "How much time am I spending thinking about this or telling this story in daily life?" Do not berate yourself, indulge frustration, or project fear into future. Notice what arises while holding onto that inner sense of "okay-ness" that resides below the surface.

5. Repeat Steps 3 and 4 with the same posture/movement. Arthritis pain often warrants response, adaptation, attention. The sensations give clues about appropriate action. As you familiarize yourself with the subtle cues of your body, breath, and mind, you gain experience that can help you understand how to respond in the moment and the future. If you come to a place where you truly feel acceptance with the challenge, does it change in any way?

You may repeat the posture or movement pattern a few times, noticing how your inner experience constantly changes. You may learn a great deal about yourself and mental habits through this practice. There is such thing as too much, however, so be careful not to ruminate. Notice when it feels like time to stop witnessing or moving, and do so. Next time you practice yoga, do your best to apply aspects of this subtle awareness. In time, it will permeate your daily life and support you in making healthy choices on a continual basis.

Self-Perception and the Role of Being Sick

When a person is ill or has been diagnosed with a life-long disease, it changes self-perception. Our health, vitality, and abilities are all included in how we tend to see ourselves. When there is a shift in our body's strength, pain, size, or activities, this can challenge our very sense of self and even precious aspects of identity. The diagnosis and symptoms of a chronic disease, such as arthritis, can change the way we think of ourselves so dramatically that we fall into a belief about a role as a sick person and lose touch with other important aspects of our identity.

From a yoga perspective, this is an example of a psychological hindrance (*klesa*), where our self-perception is attributed to external rather than internal aspects. Furthermore, there is an attachment to the old ways of being. The reality is that everyone's body is constantly changing. Once we begin to apply mindful awareness in everyday life, we come to realize that the body is more flexible on some days and more rigid others. It has less pain or more pain depending on weather, mood, nutrition choices, and many other lifestyle influences that reveal themselves over time. Some moments we feel full and others hungry. In truth, even our cells are constantly turning over, so we are literally a different body over time.

Through yoga practice, we are able to notice and respond to our ever-changing needs with greater accuracy and effectiveness, realizing that attachment to the body's particular characteristics at any given time would be futile and impractical. The moment-to-moment changes in the body occur for everyone, but they may feel more pronounced in life with arthritis. This is a challenge, but also an opportunity to discover our capacity for resilience and inner steadfastness through changing external circumstances.

Beyond applying this wisdom and awareness to the physical changes, we can also become mindful of our internal self-perceptions. When we notice the words, images, feelings, and beliefs associated with physical or emotional changes, when we identify ourselves as a sick person, we have the opportunity to intentionally change them. For example, Tina, whose story is outlined in this chapter, found that as she shifted her perspectives about her physical health and RA, she treated herself differently and her condition gradually improved. In our Yoga for Arthritis studies,[116] we found improvements in health perception and self-efficacy. In other words, students felt better able to manage their symptoms and to be in control of their overall health. The improvements that arise from changes in self-perception may not be physically dramatic, but they can elicit profound changes in mental and emotional wellbeing. A shift in perception brings a deeper sense of peace and connection to the truth of our being. And, in fact, I have found that when people change their perspective, they also start making different choices about the physical body that can also lead to powerful changes in that arena.

It is beneficial to consider why you are even in a body. When the body is completely incapacitated, important aspects of a person (kindness, creativity, humor, intelligence, etc.) continue. Apply wisdom. Acknowledge who you truly are. Your body has been changing the entire time you have had it. Consider yourself more deeply. If the body is constantly changing, who is the constant *you* that resides within it? While these questions may seem esoteric, they are at the essence of a perceptual shift.

This line of reason frames the spiritual aspects of yoga. The spirituality of yoga is not a religion; the way one engages the spiritual aspect of yoga is a personal choice. Some people use it for stress management, strength, health, or spiritual benefit. One's interaction with and understanding of yoga is self-determined. People invested in religious traditions may find resonance with yoga because its ethics and framework fit in all traditions. In this way, it is accessible to those from all faiths or no faith, or those who don't know what to believe. Swami Satchidananda, the founder of my yogic lineage, suggested that there is "one truth, many paths."[117] In other words, there are universal principles that characterize a spiritual path, and while different traditions use different strategies to get there, it all leads to a more awakened, aware, and peaceful existence. As with any spiritual tradition, yoga teaches us to be aware, live morally, and think deeply. If you do not have a current spiritual path or practice, the teachings of yoga may be a way into that side of yourself when/if those aspects of the practice resonate with you. Attune to who and what you are beyond your body and, like Tina below, appreciate that clarity may begin to inform your everyday life.

Tina's Life-Changing Shift in Perception

After Tina was diagnosed with RA, she spent years undergoing and healing from multiple surgeries. She gained weight and became inactive, which she knew affected her joints and movement abilities. While physicians recommended that she lose weight, no healthcare practitioner mentioned yoga or even any other program she could use to implement a healthier lifestyle. (If you are a clinician, please consider seeking out the resources in your community so that you can give your clients specific guidance about where they can access safe and appropriate yoga practice.)

Tina was self-reliant in finding local resources for exercise and weight loss programs for people with arthritis, which led to her participation in the Yoga for Arthritis study. One of the first benefits of yoga she noticed was a calming sense in her life. She was able to bring that focus to making improvements in the areas where she could instead of being distraught about her condition. Yoga helped Tina think of ways that she could have a positive impact and create healthy changes.

The mental change happened first, and then Tina noticed physical changes such as freedom of movement, increased energy, and generally feeling better. These benefits were self-perpetuating for Tina and made her want to practice more, which, in turn, reduced stress and increased physical benefit so that the flare-ups became less frequent. Even when flares occur, Tina is more mindful of improvements and the temporary nature of flares. She adapts her activity level accordingly and copes with the flares by being less reactive. Tina applies the wisdom of remembering that flares don't go away forever, but they do go away for a time. She is committed to doing everything she can in daily life to face challenges with grace and to work with her limitations. This includes letting go of the stress that a flare may reoccur. Instead, she "takes the upper hand" and does not let RA rule her life.

Even after being established in yoga, her RA was so bad one day that Tina could not open the tab on a can of cat food because she couldn't use her swollen, hurting hands. She witnessed herself in distress as she wept and wondered how she, a woman facing the debilitated effects of RA, could feed her beloved pets. Tina shares that the wisdom of yoga has taught her to cope with the changing limits of her body, offered humility and acceptance of limitations and personal vulnerability, and supported her in shifting her beliefs about herself and her condition.

Tina now perceives herself as having the upper hand over the disease. She is committed to enjoying her life and impacting the disease condition more than it impacts her. Even though she cannot control the flares, she made the decision to do everything possible in her life to control the RA.

Tina went from being debilitated by her disease to running 5k and 10k races competitively. Her message to others with arthritis is: "You can have a better life. It may be baby steps… It does start with moving—no matter what kind of movement, whether it's with your breath or with your body. You can have a better life… Yoga helps every body in every way."[118]

REFLECTION: LIVING A PERSONAL INTENTION

One of the fundamental books of yoga, *The Yoga Sutras*, teaches that: "When something negative arises, contemplate the opposite. This is *pratipaksa* (opposite) *bhavana* (embodied spiritual state)." This wisdom guides us to acknowledge when our thoughts and feelings are lacking discernment and breaching the primary ethical of yoga, non-harm. Lamentations, despair, and general grumpiness create harm in the brain and nervous system and, as discussed in Chapter 7, can actually exacerbate symptoms of arthritis. The intellectual *kosha* exists in the realm beyond these passing emotions. Its wisdom connects us to the true spiritual essence of our being. Giving ourselves something to hold onto, such as a meaningful intention (the "opposite" of the "negative" we experience), helps us maintain a higher awareness throughout daily life.

Cultivating an intention brings our focus away from ever-changing thoughts and experiences and connects us to the steadiness of deeper wisdom. Use the following exercise for yourself or clients to discern a personalized intention to help bring greater wisdom and ease into daily life:

1. Notice or record your negative, hurtful, or disruptive beliefs about your condition. Note the feelings and fears about the symptoms, frustrations with how it impacts your life, and the common thoughts or stories that are in your mind.

2. Acknowledge any repetitive themes. Do similar words occur? Is there a dominant emotion?

3. What feeling is the opposite of this? What soothes these habitual negative thoughts and feelings? Do not seek the linguistic antonym; rather, consider what quality neutralizes the mental/emotional pain. Consider a meaningful spiritual concept, such as peace, acceptance, self-care, nourishment, gratitude, or one of yoga's ethical principles. This is *pratipaksa bhavana*, the opposite state.

4. As you move through life, invoke this state as much as possible. You may carry or wear a symbol that helps to remind you of the kindness, connection, or love that you wish to cultivate. To be most effective, be sure to invoke this concept in response to any harmful thought/emotional patterns. This isn't to say that you don't take time sometimes to grieve the loss of health, function, or lifestyle; it's just that those moments are chosen and contained and the mind and heart are more generally set to this embodied attitude.

This new level of perception helps you operate from a perspective that is important to you. It brings greater understanding to your everyday life and helps you apply the wisdom of yoga. When you can do that, you have achieved "realized knowledge," or the kind of awareness that arises from direct experience. From there, it permeates all moments of life with your true spirit.

Summary

Yoga teaches that inside your mind, within the thinking, sensing, feeling *manomaya kosha,* lives the steady wisdom of *vijnanamaya kosha.* This layer of wisdom, or intellect, contains the ability to witness and discern the busy input from the mind. It also contains long-held beliefs. The non-judgmental observation of mindfulness practice strengthens our awareness of the intellectual *kosha.* This chapter addressed how to harness wisdom and apply it to shift the state of mind. The wisdom *kosha* is subtle and most closely aligned with our innermost essence of quietude and bliss (*anandamaya kosha*). As one connects more deeply with the subtle state of mind, there is a broader, more relaxed perspective on life. The next chapter discusses this deeper application, connecting spirituality of yoga and arthritis to daily living.

Chapter 10

SPIRITUALITY IN ARTHRITIS (*ANANDAMAYA KOSHA*)

Yoga is historically a spiritual discipline, but not everyone who practices yoga engages with its spiritual aspects. A beautiful aspect of yoga is that each person connects with whatever is essential in the moment, in alignment with individual needs and worldview. Spiritual engagement is not essential for a person to practice yoga. We might think of yoga practices as a toolbox, and perhaps the *asanas* are a hammer. If that is the only tool you ever use, you might have trouble building a house. However, you can choose to select the tools that seem most appropriate in the moment, and some tools you may choose not to use at all. For those who are not connected to the spiritual aspects of yoga, they may focus on the compelling science around breath, meditation, and sound. Either way, you should at least know what all of the tools are and how they work, so you can make informed choices about how and when you'd like to utilize them. We owe it to clients to demonstrate the efficacy of all the tools. From there, each person decides which are most useful in their unique life.

The PMK model teaches that within all the other *koshas* is the "bliss sheath," or *anandamaya kosha*. This still, quiet bliss is the essence of each of us. Yoga is not a single religion. Instead, it provides a framework for those who choose to bring their spiritual beliefs into the practice and perhaps experience relationship with Divinity more deeply, whatever that relationship may be. Conversely, those who do not believe in "something more" may be able to understand themselves and their own inner processes more deeply. This can bring a greater sense of calm, health, self-efficacy, and wellbeing in everyday life. This chapter elucidates some of the research and practices that promote spiritual wellbeing for people with arthritis.

Daily Spiritual Experiences

In 2008, I helped conduct a study that explored daily spiritual experience in people with (and without) arthritis.[119] Spirituality was identified as a strategy for coping with chronic disease. In this case, spirituality was measured through feelings of connection and support from others, thankfulness, compassion, and inner peace. It also included a sense of guidance from and trust in a Higher Power, being touched by something beautiful, and receiving comfort from community. What we found was that 80 per cent of our 99 participants reported having at least one spiritual experience most days. Those with arthritis reported significantly more daily spiritual experiences than those without arthritis. More frequent experiences were associated with increased energy and less depression in patients with arthritis.

Notably, one of the daily spiritual experiences we asked about was a sense of joy lifting them out of everyday problems. As I talked about in previous chapters, and as the PMK and BPSS models indicate, yoga impacts our consciousness and perspectives, which, in turn, has the potential to bring wellbeing to many layers of an individual. Healthcare providers are wise to ask about clients' daily spiritual experiences and emphasize them as important aspects of physical and mental health. Imbuing daily moments with meaning is a simple way to stay connected to the deepest layer of ourselves (*anandamaya kosha*) and find peace despite how the body may feel or other inclement life experiences.

Purpose and Meaning

The spiritual aspects of yoga remind us that there is a higher purpose in all things, even the pain and fatigue of arthritis. There is a concept in yoga known as *dharma*, which translates as spiritual duty or purpose. Many of our Yoga for Arthritis students profess gratitude for their disease because it has fostered better perspective and meaningful life choices. In fact, had it not been for arthritis, they may never have realized their *dharma*.

The journey through arthritis can actually enrich life, especially when it directs a focus toward personal priorities. In busy modern life, many people do not stop to contemplate their priorities. There is little time afforded to meaning and purpose. While arthritis limits opportunities in some ways, it may provide for reflection and insight. The resulting choices and richness in everyday life may lead to gratitude for all of the lessons learned through the journey. Forced to slow down, people with arthritis may take stock, re-evaluate, and reprioritise. Were it not for the diagnosis and impacts of arthritis, they may have not stopped to evaluate and live more consciously. While the challenges of the disease may not feel like a blessing, the new perspective it can foster and the new direction life sometimes takes often *do* feel like a blessing.

REFLECTION: ARTHRITIS AND YOUR *DHARMA* (PURPOSE)

There are many ways our students have gleaned specific meaning from their arthritis and taken some personal purpose from their experience of the disease. Some have chosen to make arthritis their life's work by volunteering with support organizations or working to help others with chronic conditions. In fact, approximately one third of our 200-hour Yoga for Arthritis teacher trainees have arthritis themselves; roughly two-thirds of our 500-hour trainees have arthritis. Our own individual struggles often become a beacon that guides us to our *dharma* and offers life greater meaning, while being of service to others in a unique way.

Whether you are living with arthritis, supporting someone who is, or are simply interested in this topic, it is universally important to reflect upon personal *dharma*. Answer the following questions as a means of exploring what is important and meaningful in your life, as well as acknowledging where you might uncover gratitude for the lessons that your trials have brought.

REFLECTION QUESTION #1: WHAT IS IMPORTANT TO YOU?

What do you value? If you had to narrow your priorities to the three most important things in life, what would they be? What tasks or activities are non-negotiable for you? What would you truly find painful or difficult to live without?

REFLECTION QUESTION #2: WHAT DOES IT MEAN?

Investigate why the answers to Question 1 are important. What purpose or emotion do those items give you? Which of your personal or spiritual values do they align with? What meaning do they bring, for yourself or for others?

REFLECTION QUESTION #3: WHAT ARE YOUR UNIQUE GIFTS AND EXPERIENCES?

Our *dharma* is often evident in our disposition and circumstances. What experiences have taught you great lessons in life? What challenges have you faced and transcended? What are your gifts and aptitudes? What are you keenly interested in or skilled at?

REFLECTION QUESTION #4: HOW MAY YOU CONTRIBUTE?

Where might you find opportunities in your community to put those gifts and interests to work? What organizations or groups of people would you value helping? (Note that your own inner circle of loved ones applies!) Who else might benefit from those lessons and insights? When do you feel most purposeful and engaged with society?

Allow these questions to inspire other forms of personal reflection. Throughout your day, notice when you feel most connected to who you truly are and to a sense of purpose and meaning. As you evaluate your life and how you spend your time, remain aware of your personal *dharma*. Life is more fulfilling when our habits match our purpose and intention. As the *niyama* of *tapas* teaches: patterns, or rituals, in everyday life are valuable.

Ritual: The Value of Consistency

Every culture has ritual. Some rituals exist in a religious context, while others do not. Some rituals are performed collectively as a group, while others are done alone. You may have experienced ritual in the form of cultural traditions related to the celebration of milestones or in the patterns of daily routine. When we consider how yoga might be helpful in the management of arthritic conditions, we can also think about the ritualistic aspects of yoga practice.

Ritual exists when any activity is performed in a set time, space, and/or sequence. While rituals have been performed for a myriad of reasons throughout history, it turns out that there are some measurable benefits to engaging in ritual. These benefits include better coping with both life-changing losses and mundane ones,[120] as well as reduced anxiety and brain changes that reduce the effects of failure.[121]

Yoga practices can take the form of ritual when they are performed at the same time (upon waking), in the same space (a corner of the living room), or in a particular sequence (breathing, then *asana*, then meditation). A yoga practice doesn't have to be long or elaborate to become a ritual. Perhaps you decide to take three deep breaths before entering a meeting, engage in a gratitude practice before bed, or stretch before getting up in the morning. Your yoga ritual may be the Wednesday evening class at the YMCA that you absolutely won't miss. Whatever form it takes, seeing your yoga practice as a ritual may carry its own benefits, aside from the health effects of the practices themselves. The ritualistic aspect of your practice may also help to reinforce the behavior so that it remains a consistent practice in your life for months or even years to come.

While yoga practices and other healthy behaviors can be meaningful personal rituals, another common ritual in modern life is attendance to religious services. While the ritual itself may carry health benefits, there appear to be other ways that connecting with a spiritual community could be particularly health-promoting.

Attending Church Saves Lives

Did you know that attending religious services could save your life? In fact, attending services just once per week is associated with a 33 per cent reduction in all-cause mortality,[122] which means you are less likely to die…of *anything*! Of course, we are all going to die eventually. Life, after all, is a sexually transmitted fatal condition. But people who go to church, or any other type of religious service, live longer. The next question is, of course, *why*?

First, let's just table the possibility that appealing to an omnipotent God results in answered prayers, increased favor, or other direct Divine interference. This may very well be possible, but it is impossible to measure, study, prove, or disprove…at least within the limitations of our current scientific methods. Second, we can rule out reverse causation (i.e. healthier people go to church). This is definitely true, but the study above measured many aspects of health status and health risk at baseline (when the study started) to remove those from the equation.

Sixty-five percent of reduced mortality could be explained by four factors that the scientists measured: depressive symptoms (11%), smoking (22%), social support (23%), and optimism (9%). Regarding depression, belief in a higher power can instill a sense of hope, reducing feelings of powerlessness or apathy. It's harder to feel depressed if you believe that your life is in God's hands, that you have a unique purpose, or that everything happens for a reason. Attending services also means that you are less likely to start smoking and more likely to quit. Many religions teach that the body is sacred, a temple even, and must be cared for as a creation of the Divine. Smoking is incongruous with that, meaning, it just doesn't make sense to intentionally put poison into God's divine creation. It was said by Karl Marx that "[religion] is the opium of the masses." While this was intended as a disparaging remark toward religion, it is partly true! Religion reduces pain and suffering. In this case, it could be said that religion is the anti-depressant of the long-lived.

People also tend to smoke more as a coping strategy for life challenges, and religion has a built-in set of coping strategies that otherwise equip participants to manage those challenges. That doesn't necessarily make it easy to quit, but it might be easier not to start, and the social support and resources available through a congregation can help with quitting. The same might be true of other unhealthy habits—whether or not you are doing them when you start attending, going to services changes your health behaviors for the better.

Social support, the strongest element measured, affects health in countless ways. Belonging to a community provides its own sense of meaning and purpose, aside from any religious beliefs. Attending weekly services makes it likely that other congregants know your name, ask about your family, and give you a smile or a hug. All of this is good for your health. More practically speaking, this community provides a network of support and assistance. If you need a ride to the doctor, someone might volunteer. If you are ill, someone might visit or bring you a hot meal. If you have fallen on hard times, someone might know of a place you can stay or they might provide warm clothes for your family. This community also serves as a social network. Someone from your congregation might help you get an appointment at an overscheduled doctor's office; they might connect you with a lawyer who can help settle your deceased mother's estate; they might offer financial recommendations that help you plan for a comfortable retirement. A community like this expands your social connections, your access to resources, and all the while lets you know that someone cares about how you are doing and is willing to offer a kindness when needed.

Lastly, optimism is higher among those who attend religious services. Certainly, it is easier to be optimistic if you believe that you are chosen, saved, favored, and/ or will be rewarded in the afterlife as a result of your good deeds, faith, struggles, or birthright. Furthermore, the content of the religious service, be it hymns, chants, call-and-response, a sermon, or communal silence, can uplift, restore hope, and send you back out into the sunshine (or moonlight) to greet the day with a different perspective.

What does this have to do with yoga or even with arthritis? It actually has to do with both! Yoga can be practiced alone, but it is often practiced in group settings. In that way, yoga is a communal practice. While some may think of yoga as simply exercise or stress reduction, the initial purpose of yoga, and even its very translation, is about connection with Divine Source, whatever you might call it (God, Allah, Universe, Higher Self, etc.). If you get still and quiet and pay attention to your experience, you might notice something in your knee, you might notice something in your mind, or you might notice something in your soul. After all, we are spiritual beings having a human experience and your soul doesn't head out for a coffee break when you walk into a yoga class.

So, while yoga isn't a religion and yoga class isn't a religious service, it could have some of the same benefits that attending church can have. In fact, if you do have a strong religious faith, you probably bring that faith with you into yoga practice. You might pray during the silent meditation, set an intention related to your beliefs, choose a mantra with meaning, or thank God for your body and all it can do. Unfortunately, there has been some confusion that suggests yoga is antithetical to a particular religion, but since yoga is not a religion, it is a set of practices that can be experienced through any religious lens, or even none at all. A yoga community, or *sangha*, can also provide many of the benefits that a church community provides, in terms of social support, social capital, and social networks. We know that yoga reduces depressive symptoms and that yogis are less likely to smoke and might also be more optimistic. Imagine how much longer you might live if you go to religious services *and* yoga class!

People living with arthritis experience challenges that may be particularly well suited to the benefits of communal spiritual practice. Arthritis is associated with higher rates of depression,[123] likely due to both inflammatory processes and the challenges of chronic pain. Smoking increases arthritis symptoms and is even a major risk factor for onset of RA.[124] People living with disability, fatigue, and other challenges of arthritis can benefit from the support of community members, especially during flares or in recovery from surgery. It can sometimes be difficult to feel optimistic when living with a chronic disease, so anything that may help with reframing the situation and feeling more positive is probably a good idea. In fact, in our research examining the daily spiritual experiences of people living with arthritis and those without,[125] people living with arthritis had more daily spiritual experiences than those without arthritis. It is possible that spirituality is one way to help manage the pain and uncertainty of life with arthritis and those who had more spiritual experiences also had lower levels of depression and more energy. Another study showed that people with more spiritual experiences have better mood and better self-rated health, regardless of their disease status, physical function, or age.[126]

If you have a religious community, thank them for extending your life! If you don't attend very often, consider going a little bit more. If you don't have a religious community, consider finding one that feels like a good fit with your beliefs. No matter what your relationship to religion, take your yoga practice outside of the house when you can. Find a yoga class and a yoga community that is a fit with your physical abilities and your spiritual leanings that can help you to live a longer, happier life.

REFLECTION: RITUALS FOR HEALTH

This exercise supports you in changing unhealthy habits at their source. It is inspired by concepts in the book *Motivational Interviewing*. You may think of it as applying that *niyama* of surrender (*ishvara pranidhana*). You or your clients may repeat this process for each aspect of lifestyle that may be limiting health, such as nutrition, boundaries, relationships, working, movement, sleep, fun, etc.

1. Select one habit that you want to change, like eating late at night, taking on too much or saying yes when you mean no.

2. List or draw a picture to represent the effects of this habit on various aspects of your life. Acknowledge both the benefits and the harms that it brings.

3. What will you lose if you are no longer making this choice? How will it harm you to no longer have this behavior? What will you miss? Are there other—healthier—ways you can meet those same needs?

4. What is the underlying need that it is meeting or the belief that feeds this unhealthy pattern?

5. What is the first step toward changing it? Answer this from a personal, not necessarily a rational, point of view. What might be your first step is not the first step someone else would need. If possible, break down that first step into even smaller pieces. What are parts one, two, and three of that first step to change?

6. When the pattern repeats itself (i.e. temptation, craving, relapse), what do you need to remember? How will you remind yourself that it is important to neutralize it more fully? You may create a mantra, have an image of a healthier self, or call a supportive friend who encourages you to become healthier.

7. Appreciate yourself for taking this action. List some concrete, healthy self-care activities that help you feel loved or relaxed.

When we investigate the source of a behavior and acknowledge the complex reasons we engage in it, this clarity helps us let go. Curiosity and acceptance are important attitudes in this process of surrendering (*ishvara pranidhana*) unhealthy behaviors. Observe your answers and choices calmly and enjoy the process of self-inquiry and change!

New York Yoga for Arthritis Community

A drop-in Yoga for Arthritis class runs regularly in New York. A wonderful *sangha* of teachers work with diverse attendance of people with OA, RA, and chronic pain. The students are different each week and the teachers are also on rotation, so there is a great mix of people showing up in that community. This is different from the classes at Johns Hopkins, where the same community of people gathers for eight weeks and learns from the same teacher. Relationships are built in New York, too, but it is not the same because of the continually shifting teachers and participants. This diversity makes it a terrific laboratory for mentoring Yoga for Arthritis teachers as they rotate through classes over time, gaining practical experience with a range of abilities. The teachers learn a great deal from the many people they instruct and are also mentored by senior Yoga for Arthritis staff. Similarly, students are exposed to various nuances of practice as each teacher brings an exclusive flavor.

Students arriving for the first time complete a brief intake card. This card notes physical regions of concern and other relevant notes about students' health and practice. Cards are stored in locked box and each time a student attends, relevant updates or changes and specific symptoms are noted. Students sign a waiver allowing this intake card to be shared amongst the Yoga for Arthritis teachers so they may remain apprised of students' progress and other updates. The intake cards function as an ongoing assessment for as long as attendance continues; thus, each class is guided by what is happening with each student. There are opportunities for students to share with each other and teachers to connect with each student.

These check-ins at the beginning of class, along with other conversations the students have with one another, are some of what makes Yoga for Arthritis classes especially beneficial. In many cases, regular yoga classes don't serve the purpose a Yoga for Arthritis class is asked to serve. As in the New York class, there is a common experience among students and they can share how yoga supports them with the physical, mental, and spiritual aspects of arthritis. In the BPSS model, these kinds of classes contribute to social health. Students have an opportunity to share the difficulties of their experiences or gain inspiration from others' similar journeys. They can share helpful information and support each other as students speak to specific solutions to their conditions. The role of relaxation and parasympathetic engagement in immune function, for example, or how the synovial fluid of the joints relates soothes arthritis symptoms. They may share how a shift in perspective transformed a former stress into an opportunity for compassion or peace. Social isolation is common for people struggling with a chronic condition and Yoga for Arthritis classes offer a community and many opportunities for connection.

POSTURE: NEW YORK YOGA FOR ARTHRITIS SAMPLE PRACTICE

Even though social connection is a key benefit of the Yoga for Arthritis classes at the Integral Yoga Institute in New York City, the beginning of class is set up to cultivate privacy. Lights are dim and participants rest on a soft "mat sandwich" consisting of a blanket between two yoga mats. Because the floors are hardwood, this allows a "sticky" support on top and bottom but also sufficient cushioning for sensitive bodies.

The class begins in Reclining Bound Angle, a restorative pose. In this pose, a bolster is placed at an angle, supported by two blocks at different heights. The student rests back on the bolster, soles of the feet together, with support under the knees, such as rolled blankets or blocks (Figure 10.1).

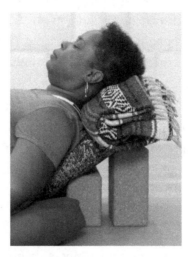

Figure 10.1: Supported Reclining Position

While this pose is incredibly relaxing, it can also feel vulnerable in a room of relative strangers. Because of this, the mats are placed in a herringbone orientation, so that no one is directly facing another student. Some students also prefer to be covered with a blanket for warmth and/or security. There is also a chair behind the bolster set-up for later in the class. This beginning ritual is established and experienced students in New York know to come in and assume the relaxation pose. A great peacefulness fills the room as people mentally and physically prepare themselves for class via relaxation.

During this personal relaxation, teachers perform quiet individual check-ins with students about their condition and how they are feeling, while others in the class are doing something constructive: restoring themselves. This helps to reduce any stress or tension that accumulated in the effort to get to class, which can be substantial in New York City, and can impact pain, physical function, and mindfulness during class. As the class begins, students then benefit from the mobilizing and stabilizing benefits of yoga. The following describes the typical New York Yoga for Arthritis class. Feel free to give this a try on your own. Remember to consult the Appendix for variations on the postures listed in the following class sequence.

Just as the teachers check in with each student, you may check in with yourself. Note changes in chronic areas of pain, swelling, or immobility. Witness your thoughts and acknowledge your emotions as they move through you. Feel yourself distancing from everyday stress and mental busyness as you connect to something deeper within. This may feel like a sense of stillness, peace, love, or general "okay-ness."

Once the teacher has checked in with each student it is time for group instruction. Teachers guide the class through breath awareness, which you may practice now by simply noticing your breath. You may deepen this, just as they do in New York, by placing more emphasis on extending the exhale. During this time, teachers affirm the individual nature of practice and ensure inclusiveness. Right now, appreciate your individuality and remind yourself that you can practice in whatever way you want, following the body's messages as your guide to safety and comfort. Notice any places where your body is making contact with a prop or the floor. Allow yourself to let go and be the supported. Deepen those points of contact and let yourself sink in.

Relaxation and safety broaden as teachers remind the class (or you remind yourself) to let go of day, the stress of getting to class, and any negativity or frustration that they may be carrying. This cueing helps shift from a narrow, manomaya (mentally) informed perspective to a broader vijnanamaya (wisdom) and even anandamaya (spiritual) acknowledgement of life. Stresses pass and are rarely relevant for long. This reminder helps students (and you) come to a more relaxed state and dial back the sympathetic (stress) response of the nervous system.

Continue breathing deeply, setting the mind to the good feelings of practice, and generate heat in your hands by rubbing the palms together rapidly. As you do that, consider any places in the body that could benefit from a little bit of extra loving kindness. Once the hands are warm, take the palms to those parts of the body asking for some attention. Let the heat dissipate in that location as though it could bring healing energy to the body. You may even perform gentle rubbing or massage. Repeat that process with generating heat between the palms, this time bringing them to another part of the body that would like attention.

As *asana* practice begins, students are given practical suggestions around physical safety and care, such as trusting the cues of their bodies and not overextending. Modify practice as much as possible for comfort and ease. A second level of practical suggestions include reminders of self-acceptance, appreciation for the body and all it can do, and choosing a calm state of mind.

Begin movement in this supported position by mobilizing every joint. This releases synovial fluids to help lubricate each joint. Keeping the body in its supported position, begin by gently turning the head from side to side, allowing it to roll from one ear to the other, supported by the bolster. Roll the shoulders next, feeling the shoulderblades slide along the support of the bolster, while allowing room for the shoulders to move. Roll the wrists, wiggle the fingers, and create larger movements of the arms before allowing them to rest.

Now let the knees fall gently over to the left. You may want to take the support that was under your right knee and bring it between the knees as they fall to the left. You might choose to remove the support from under the left knee if that feels okay. Spend a few moments breathing into this twist, dropping the right shoulder into the bolster, and perhaps turning the head to the right if that feels fine. As you are ready, gently take the knees over to the right for a few breaths on the other side. When you are ready, remove the props from around the knees and move between these two twisting poses more dynamically, as though your legs were windshield wipers moving in perfect unison. As you finish this movement, bring the knees up to center with the feet planted on the floor.

Still relaxing into the bolster, slide the right heel away from you, as if pushing something away with the sole of your foot, and then draw the heel back in and plant the foot on the floor. Try this on the other side and alternate between sides, noticing how the knees, hips, and ankles are aligned as you move. Do they follow a straight line of alignment or go off track, wobbling in and out of place? Do they move around certain points on the line consistently, like a path around a tree? Do they act as an integrated part of the leg? Pay attention to the sensations and relationships of hips, knees, and feet. Now extend both legs for a moment. Rotate the ankles. Point and flex the feet/toes.

As you are ready, roll to one side, coming off of the bolster to bring yourself to a seated position. You may want to sit up on the bolster with support under the knees. Bring yourself into a position that allows the spine to be upright. Close the eyes here and notice how the body feels after moving in all directions and with each joint. This is a nice time in the class to set an intention for focus, to practice some deep diaphragmatic breathing, and perhaps to engage in a meaningful chant.

Cat-Cow is the next sequence, bringing more movement into the whole spine. This can be done in a seated position, or you might choose to come onto hands and knees with a folded blanket under the knees for extra cushioning. If done on hands and knees, other options can be added, such as looking over one shoulder toward the hip, extending one limb or opposite limbs together (ie. right arm and left leg). If you have done Cat-Cow from a seated position, it is nice to extend the legs into a Staff Pose for a moment and feel the energy of the body's long lines.

Move the floor props out of the way, excluding a folded blanket by the chair behind you. Turn to face the chair and with the knees on the blanket, place the hands on the chair for support and bring yourself up to standing. Come around behind the chair for standing and balancing poses, moving the chair forward on the mat to make room as needed.

Come to Mountain Pose (*Tadasana*) behind the chair with feet a hip distance apart, holding onto the chair for stability if you choose. Eyes can be open or closed. Lift the toes and set them down consciously to feel grounded. You may imagine the feet growing roots into the earth as the legs grow upward like strong trunks. Knees are soft; belly moves with the breath; spine is long and sweeping, neck reaching into the base of the skull as the eyes gaze forward, chin parallel to the floor. You may insert one of the Sun Salutation variations from Chapters 5 or 11 here, then proceed to the next few standing poses.

Shift your weight from side to side and feel your center of gravity shift. This helps you learn to adapt to various balancing challenges and can help prevent falls. Place a tall-backed chair on your yoga mat in front of you to support your balance. Allow the weight to shift to your right leg as you prepare to balance on one foot. Open your left leg to the side, rotating the hip, and place the left heel on the right ankle or calf. Do not press against the side of the knee, which puts excess strain on the joint. You may hold the chair, bring hands to hips, out to the sides like a tightrope walker, or overhead. Allow yourself to adjust and adapt—

those wobbles help you become more secure and balanced! Repeat Tree Pose (*Vrkasana*) on the other side then return to Mountain Pose.

Bring the feet wide apart and ensure that the hips turn out comfortably without creating much twist in the knee. For most people, pointing the toes out at a 45-degree angle helps maintain alignment. As you bend the knees, ensure they move over the ankles but not beyond them. Press the outside ("pinky" toe side) of the foot into the earth to help the knees stay open and aligned. Hands may rest on the chair, hips, or shoulders, or raise the elbows to the sides, in line with the shoulders, and bend the elbows so the palms face forward. This is Goddess Pose (*Deviasana*). Breathe a sense of groundedness and empowerment.

Bring legs hip-width apart again. Hinge from the hips and surrender into a Forward Fold (*Uttanasana*). Feel yourself letting go of tension. You can bring hands to chair seat, thighs, or support the elbows against the knees. Allow the back of the neck to lengthen and release. To come out of the posture, roll the spine up. Your hands can climb up the legs or chair while the abdominal muscles also support the back as you rise up. Once standing, hold the back of the chair and create a small backbend by making space between navel and ribs, lifting the chest forward and up. Be sure to keep hips stable. Find Mountain Pose again and feel the effects of these standing poses.

Now come to sitting in the chair with a blanket on the seat as needed. Ankles are beneath the knees, knees aligned with the hip joints. Stabilize through the seat, lengthen the torso, and find your Seated Mountain. When ready, begin revolving to the right for a seated spinal twist, moving from the base of the spine up through the crown of the head. Once you've moved into a comfortable twist, you can hold onto the back of the chair with the right hand, bring the left hand to the right leg or bring the arms into any other comfortable position. Be sure not to pull or force a deepening in this pose, but simply allow it to be gentle and easy. Repeat the twist on the left side. You may perform this modified seated twist again before moving on to the next posture.

After the twist, take a moment to notice how the body feels. Give yourself the opportunity to do any movement that feels like a good idea. This may be a big stretch, your favorite pose, or something that just feels right in the moment. When you are ready, return to Seated Mountain and take stock of how you feel. If you set an intention earlier in class, bring your awareness back to that intention.

From here, cross the ankles or bring the soles of the feet together. Take the arms around the back of the body to hold opposite wrist or bring the hands to the low back. Tuck the chin toward the chest and bring your focus inward toward the body's core and your inner essence. In this variation of Symbol of Yoga Post (*Yoga Mudra*), seal in the benefits of this whole-person practice, connecting to your spirit in this inward-focused posture. Acknowledge the benefits of practice, the many things your body does for you each day, sending it appreciation, along with anything else in life you are thankful for. After a few even breaths, release a tall seated position and prepare for final relaxation. You may choose to do this in a seated position, perhaps with the chair at the wall so that your head can have some support. You might want to come to the floor, lying on your back, or even rest your lower legs on the seat of the chair.

Once you have found a comfortable position for relaxation, supported by props as needed, allow the body to sink into the pose and let go of any muscular tension. You might consider tensing each part of the body and then allowing it to release, which can help the muscles to relax more. Scan the body from toes to head, encouraging each body part to relax. Allow the breath to deepen and soften. Let the mind rest in calm and stillness. Let yourself just be for a few minutes of peace.

As you are ready, gently roll onto one side and come to a seated position on the floor or on the chair, perhaps with props for support. Notice any effects this gentle practice may have had on your body, energy, thoughts, feelings, and inner self.

The class finishes with a short meditation practice. Sitting upright, allow yourself to deepen the breath. As you relax and your mind clears a bit more, focus on an uplifting word, sensation, or image. If you mind wanders from it, simply bring it back with compassion and understanding. After a few minutes of meditation, you may choose to close with a chant, song, or prayer. Open the eyes and return your awareness to the space around you and to your everyday life. Carry the ease and awareness of practice with you into your daily actions and interactions.

Pam's Story

Pam, like many people with arthritis, lived without a proper diagnosis for a long time. She thought she had OA, but it turns out she had RA. What that means is her RA was completely unmanaged and in constant flare for many years without her knowing any differently. She lived with the pain, fatigue, swelling, and other symptoms of systemic arthritis as if it were a part of life. Eventually she received the correct diagnosis. Pam was dedicated to her yoga practice but required a great deal of modification due to the severe manifestation of her disease. The Yoga for Arthritis community is an accepting one, where each person is encouraged to work with her/his own body and select the appropriate intensity.

Students in the Yoga for Arthritis classes are aware of one another but do not judge or compare. In this *sangha,* students follow internal as well as external guidance and do not expect to look like anyone else in the room as they each engage in their own best practice. It was no secret that Pam required a great deal of assistance to move from the floor back to a standing position. In her first class, I nonchalantly offered a hand of support. It continued like that for several classes, twice per week, once each class. Without stopping the flow of my verbal instruction to the class, I would walk over to Pam and offer my support.

About halfway through the eight-week program, I stuck to the routine of reaching out my hand to Pam and she refused it. She was on one knee, with the other foot on the floor, and she politely waved off my assist. "No," she said. "I'm going to do it myself."

At this point, the rest of the room was already in Mountain Pose and Pam's words drew their attention. I did not move on with the class, lest we leave Pam behind, so I stood…and watched…and waited. The whole class stood…and watched…and waited. Time seemed to move very slowly. I was concerned for Pam, with so much attention on her, and for her classmates in this potentially awkward situation. As Pam struggled to position herself and engage her muscles, the rest of the class waited on.

Slowly and deliberately, Pam made her way to standing. The effort was visible on her face; the exertion showed in her shaking muscles. Eventually, she stood like the rest of the class. Once she arrived in Mountain Pose, the whole room broke into applause! It is a great testament to the social support that comes from a class setting. The Yoga for Arthritis community is different from some mainstream classes that do not foster community or individual approaches to practice. That group, only acquainted a few weeks, was genuinely full of pride for Pam's accomplishment and saw their own potential and healing in her journey. The yoga strengthened Pam. Witnessing that strength and receiving support may give the entire community a little more strength for whatever they may face in their journey through life with arthritis.

Chanting

When we conducted the Yoga for Arthritis study at Johns Hopkins, it was based on my training as a teacher of Integral Yoga. I had just recently completed my 200-hour yoga teacher training and developed the program based on how I was taught to teach yoga. I modified many elements of the practice based on my experience with arthritis patients, but I didn't remove any components. As such, it represented a comprehensive yoga practice, including centering, breathwork, moving sequences, held poses of all kinds, relaxation, meditation, philosophy, and chanting. When I was asked to help replicate the study at NIH, the Institutional Review Board asked us to remove all "spiritual" elements of the practice. Now, my thoughts about the impossibility of such a proposition is discussed elsewhere in this book. Nonetheless, chanting was one of those elements deemed too spiritual for inclusion. This is not uncommon. Chanting is often left out of yoga classes and interventions, which I really think is a disservice to the students and the practice itself.

Chanting has been part of almost every religious and spiritual tradition throughout history and across the globe. It combines the benefits of controlled breathing with sound vibration and meaning, whether through a shared experience or solo practice. These three elements have the opportunity to impact mind-body-spirit in a variety of ways. For example, a study that used repetitive chanting of a meaningful word was associated with a tempered response to negative experiences.[127] In other words, chanting helped reduce the brain impact of encountering something negative. It can help to keep us steadier in the face of challenges, perhaps including the challenges of life with a chronic, painful disease. Not surprisingly, chanting is also associated with improved pulmonary outcomes.[128] Improved pulmonary function can also impact the heart, which may be more challenged for individuals with arthritis of any form, for a variety of reasons (i.e. inflammation, obesity, reduced physical activity). Additionally, chanting alters the brain's limbic system,[129] which is associated with emotional reactivity and the formation of new memories about past experiences. So, chanting might help change how we feel about a situation and even what we think about it. That's powerful stuff!

However, we shouldn't disregard that chanting has a cultural context and may create discomfort or alienation, depending on how it is presented. Since most religious traditions have some history of chanting, it is possible to incorporate chants from any tradition into a yoga practice. For yoga that happens in a community with shared cultural and religious traditions, this may work well. Bringing in chants from an individual's spiritual or cultural tradition may also work in one-on-one yoga therapy practice. The meaning attributed to the chant by the person chanting it may be more important than the nuance of the sound vibration, although that has not been explored scientifically. In diverse communities, a more universally-accepted sound might work best. In some situations, I have taken the sound of *Om* and broken it down into three separate parts (Ah, Oh, Mm) to retain its vibrational qualities without the cultural context. We "chant" three times, sighing each of these sounds. It requires a deep breath in and a long, slow exhale, which turns off the stress response while also creating the resonance of sound that may have its own impact on body, mind, and spirit. You might also consider incorporating secular song or verse that has meaning relevant to the goals of yoga practice. Because songs imprint powerful memories and emotions, use caution and care if/when incorporating them into yoga practice.

In several religious traditions, the word is considered sacred. In modern life, we often use language carelessly without regard for the powerful impact it might have on those who hear it, but also on those who speak it. When I suggest using chants from other traditions, I do that in order to make the practice accessible and acceptable to diverse audiences who may benefit from it. It is important to note that the chants of yoga each have a different intention and are ascribed different associations and effects in tradition and text. For those who feel comfortable chanting in Sanskrit, there is a lot to explore within that tradition. Since Sanskrit is no longer a spoken language, there is something beautiful about the preservation of its use without the trappings of modern common discourse.

Consider this an invitation to play around with sound. Notice how different sounds can be felt in different parts of the body. Notice how it feels to chant a meaningless sound or a powerful word. Notice the effect of sound vibration on the feeling of a room, even after it is no longer audible. When designing a yoga practice for health and healing, don't reflexively remove chanting from the formula. If well-chosen, you might be surprised by the impact it has.

Summary

This chapter discussed the benefits of spiritual connection as we explored material manifestations of *anandamaya kosha*. This still, quiet bliss is the essence of each of us. Each practitioner is free to personalize the quality of engagement and offer an individual meaning and purpose to practice. Physical, energetic, mental, and intellectual ease are required in order to connect to that bliss state. This does not mean that we must be pain-free in order to experience the deepest layer of ourselves. What we do with our wisdom (*vijnanamay kosha*) and perspectives has the greatest impact on our spiritual connection. What we do for the mind (*manomaya kosha*) is powerful as it sets the stage for a clear intellect. What we do for the energy (*pranamaya kosha*) and body (*annamaya kosha*) is also important as they house those deeper layers. When we are at peace and spiritually connected, there is a greater connection to true wellbeing, even in times when the body is not healthy. *Anandamaya kosha* feeds the other layers and, when we take time to quiet ourselves and connect, provides a frame for uplifted beliefs, emotions, thoughts, and lifestyle. The following part of the book provides you with sequences you can incorporate into everyday life to create a healthy ritual of movement and awareness.

PART III

YOGA THERAPY PRACTICES FOR ARTHRITIS

This final part of the book is practical. It offers you a series of practices you may play with at home or recommend to your clients. You could also use these sequences as a frame and work with your yoga therapist or healthcare provider to customize the movements, breathing practices, and visualizations for your unique needs. Each practice includes intention-setting and other subtle practices such as breathing exercises, relaxation, visualization, or meditation, as these are highly important parts of yoga. Please be sure to consult the Appendix for variations on postures and adaptive patterns that help you get the most out of the practices while maintaining a healthy approach that suits you.

Chapter 11

YOGA THERAPY AT HOME

Throughout the book, we have offered sample posture, breathing, relaxation, and meditation practices. Any of these will fit nicely into a daily practice. The following chapter provides instructions for establishing a safe home practice that will help with managing arthritis symptoms. Be sure to check out the Appendix for pose modifications that address varying levels of challenge and adaptation. Images are also included there. Stay connected to your body's messages and a meaningful intention at all times. Remember that your practice is your own, and as long as you are following a few basic guidelines of safety and sequencing, you are free to play, adapt, edit and incorporate as you wish. Home practice is the gift you give yourself whenever you do it. The benefits of home practice can (sometimes surprisingly) seep into all five *koshas* and through every area of life: biological, psychological, social, and spiritual.

Sequencing Guidelines

There are some general guidelines that can help you create your own home practice. The basic sequencing for many yoga classes includes:

1. Centering—This may be intention-setting, contemplative awareness, chanting, deep breathing, or some other form of personal reflection that brings you into awareness of the present moment and into a proper mindset for practice.

2. Warm-Up—In a Yoga for Arthritis class, these are simple movements that help to lubricate the joints, decrease stiffness, and warm up the muscles to prepare for deeper practice (see the sequence later in this chapter for an example).

3. *Asanas*—A series of poses to foster health and wellbeing are combined in a predictable sequence that addresses strength, flexibility, and balance of the whole body. Poses can be held for varying lengths of time, depending on your experience, intention for practice, characteristics of the pose, and your needs on that day.

4. Any complete sequence will involve at least one posture from each pose category: forward bend, backward bend, side bend, twist, and upward reaching. These postures may be standing, seated, reclined, balancing, or inverted. Try to think about the poses in pairs, so that each movement gets an equal and opposite movement to maintain a sense of balance in the body.

5. *Pranayama*—Breathing practices amplify the benefits of *asanas*. Movement can be connected with the breath throughout yoga practice. In some poses, this means moving one direction on an inhale and the opposite direction on an exhale (though you can always adapt these patterns, too). Some teachers also instruct students to hold a pose for a particular number of breaths. Independent of the *asanas,* there is often another set of breathing practices during class to invigorate or calm the body and mind.

6. Relaxation—Near the end of practice, some type of relaxation is recommended, ideally for between 4 and 12 minutes. This is usually done in *Savasana* or Corpse Pose. The purpose of this relaxation is to absorb the tension-reducing benefits of the *asanas*, so that a sense of calm and ease will carry over from the practice into the rest of the day. It also relates to the original purpose of *hatha* practice: relaxing the body so that it can remain quiet for meditation.

7. Meditation—This is a time to quiet and focus the mind, relieving it of the unnecessary clutter and trivial thoughts that stream in and out during the

day. This discipline of the mind can provide relief from daily stresses and may also foster spiritual awareness or experiences. Meditation changes the brain, which can alter pain and coping. Your meditation can have any focus, such as the breath, an image, an idea or affirmation, a sound, or a personal prayer. You can perform meditation while standing or in any seated position. If you are not able to stand or sit comfortably, lying down is fine, too. If you can't stay awake in a reclined meditation posture, your body likely needs the rest.

8. Acknowledgement—Before leaving the practice space, thankfully acknowledge the changes practice may have allowed, however subtle. Feel appreciation for yourself, cultivating the discipline and treating yourself to healthy routines. Secure the benefits and intention so that they remain with you as you transition into everyday life. Remember them throughout the day.

Experiment with the sequences in this chapter. Each one is designed to follow the above guidelines and includes a sample relaxation, breathing practice, and meditative focus. You can mix and match these final components for a personalized experience each time. Incorporate favorite postures from your own yoga class or yoga therapy sessions. If you decide to alter the pose sequences, please be sure to include all the posture categories listed above and always move with care and ease. Sequences performed in a chair are beneficial for people with limited mobility, who feel unsafe or unsteady on their feet, or who do not have the strength/energy for a standing practice. If you have any questions about what poses and movements are safe and appropriate for you, be sure to consult with a health provider for guidance. Above all, practice in the way that feels best for you. Enjoy!

POSTURE, RELAXATION, BREATHING, CONCENTRATION: JOINT LUBRICATION

This sequence is an excellent way to warm up before performing any other practices in this or the next chapter. It helps "lubricate" the joints and get synovial fluid moving. Practice it anytime you are feeling stiff or want to prevent stiffness. These simple movements mobilize the joints in sequence. Begin seated away from the back of the chair so that you are able to support your own spine, if possible. Check that the thigh bones are parallel to each other and the ankles are straight below the knees, with feet flat on the floor (or a prop as needed). Sit up tall, creating length in the spine, and imagine that your head floats on top of the spine. Soften your gaze so it is relaxed and not a hard stare. Allow your breath to deepen and soften. Notice if your mind is distracted and bring it into the present moment:

1. Neck: Keep the rest of the back tall, lengthen the neck by dropping the chin toward the chest then lengthening the head upward slightly to open the throat. With slow control, make a nodding "yes" movement, bringing the head only high enough to gaze where the wall and ceiling meet (not dropping the head back to look at the ceiling above you). Next, tilt the head to the right, then left, moving each ear towards its shoulder *without* lifting the shoulder towards the ear. You may coordinate these movements with breath, inhaling one way and exhaling the other. From center, twist the neck gently by looking only slightly over one shoulder then the other without moving the torso. Do not force these stretches; allow for soft, fluid, easy movement that stays within a comfortable range.

2. Thoracic Spine:

   a. Backward/Forward Spinal Action: Repeat the movement sequence above, layering in the movement of the middle back. Nod the head and bring the upper torso along in a sort of Cat-Cow action. You may move the arms front and back as you go, sliding them along the thighs in order to elaborate the movement, coordinating with the breath so that you round on the exhale and open the chest on the inhale.

   b. Simple Side Stretch: Sit up tall, lengthening one arm alongside the chair and then the other so that the spine bends both ways. Notice how you can stay strong on both sides of the body at the same time, as the low ribs get closer to the hip on one side and further away on the other side. Feel this contracting and opening on opposite sides. Breathe with the movement, perhaps exhaling and you go to each side and inhaling as you return to center.

   c. Seated Twist: Again, sit up nice and tall. Let one hand slide toward the knee on one leg while the other hand slides toward the hip on the other leg. Allow this movement to continue through the torso, creating a gentle twist in each direction. Create a smooth, continuous movement through the upper torso and neck as you twist gently from side to side.

Consider exhaling as you twist and inhaling as you return to center. As your breath remains smooth, so the movement will also remain fluid.

3. Lumbar Spine:

    a. Repeat the movements from above, layering the action of the lumbar spine into the postures. Nod the head, round/arch the back, and roll front to back on the sitz bones at the base of the pelvis. These are the pointing bones you can feel through the gluteal tissue. You are performing a full seated Cat-Cow, making a continuous forward and backward bending movement. You might involve the arms even more so that the elbows bend and straighten, allowing the movement to be even larger.

    b. As you perform the side bend, experience the length and compression at the waistline. Consider adding the arms, holding onto the chair with one hand for support and extending the other arm overhead, reaching as you bend.

    c. Sitting up tall, create a fuller twist, imagining the rotation through the cervical, thoracic, and lumbar spine. Repeat on the other side. Avoid pulling or forcing, and keep the movement within a comfortable range. You may move through this action a few times.

4. Shoulders:

    a. Roll the shoulders around one way, then the other. You may draw a spiral in the air, starting with very small movements then making them bigger or decreasing your big shoulder rolls into tiny spirals.

    b. Roll the shoulders, alternating one at a time in each direction. Notice how the spine and ribs are also a part of this shoulder roll. If you feel discomfort or "crunching," simply make the movement smaller or slower, or adjust in any other way that makes the movement more comfortable.

5. Elbows: With the arms out to the sides or in front of you, bend and straighten at the elbows. Play around with how slow and how large you make that movement. You can also rotate the lower arms in and out so

that the palms turn toward ceiling and floor. See if you can perform these movements without moving the upper arms or shoulders.

6. Wrists: Hold the arms in front of you and flex/extend your wrists so the fingers point up and then down. Only do this within a comfortable range, so it is fine to keep the movement small. Now roll the wrists one way then the other. Try circling them in the same direction as each other and then in opposite directions.

7. Fingers: Lengthen the arms alongside the chair. Stretch your fingers long toward the floor, then create space as the fingers stretch wide away from each other. Bring the hands onto your lap and wiggle your fingers as if you were playing the piano. Lift the hands off of your lap and take each finger toward the thumb one at a time, whether it touches or not, to get the bones moving through the hands. Now spread the palms wide and let the hands close a few times, as if you were making gentle fists then stretching. Again, it is not important whether you can make a fist, only that you are stretching, strengthening, and mobilizing the hands in a variety of ways.

8. Arm Improvisation: Move your arms however you choose! Swim a front crawl or backstroke, dance the arms or create expressive shapes with your upper limbs. Allow your torso, neck, and head to play along. Feel the lubrication of these joints and allow yourself to stretch out any lingering stiffness.

9. Toes: Leave the soles of the feet on the floor as you wiggle the toes, reaching them out of the balls of the feet. Spread the toes wide and then press them into the floor. See if you can control the toes independently by moving each one in sequence. This can help to support improved balance.

10. Feet/Ankles: Rock back and forth across the soles of the feet, so the toes and then heels lift off the floor. Feel the movement of all those tiny bones in the feet, as well as noticing how the ankles move with this action. You can play a brain game by lifting right toes and lowering left heel, then trading sides. Stamp the feet quickly and gently on the floor. Take the feet out to the sides and back in a few times. Roll the ankles in each direction.

11. Hips: Slide back in the chair so that you are supported by the chair back. Sit tall and grip the sides of the chair for support. Keep the feet planted on

the floor and then lift right leg on the inhale, lower on the exhale. Repeat on the left side. Keep the thigh on the chair and notice the engagement of your thigh muscles as you go. Now try a sequence: 1) lift the leg; 2) draw the knee in toward the torso; 3) extend the leg out; and 4) lower it down. Be sure you continue to sit up tall on the sitz bones and breathe with each movement. Connect with those large muscles that are so important for maintaining independence. Lift the right leg with the knee bent and draw thigh in small circles within the hip socket. Repeat on the other side. Slide to the right in your chair, holding onto the chair seat with your left hand. Slide the right leg back alongside the chair, lowering the knee toward the floor. This should be stretching the muscles in the front of the hip that are often tight from a lot of sitting. You can also stretch the right arm overhead and even reach left in a side stretch. Repeat on the other side. Shake the legs out however feels good.

12. Movement Completion: Move anything else that requires additional movement. Revisit any of the above actions again and notice how the joints respond differently at the end of practice compared to when you first engaged them. Consider a stretch, twist, wiggle, or shake. Acknowledge your increased freedom of movement and celebrate yourself for engaging in this practice.

13. Relaxation: Settle into the support of the chair back, perched tall on your sitz bones, allowing the natural sweep of your spine. Even though you are holding your head up, it feels easy due to its alignment with your neck and torso. You may move your head slightly forward and back to find the place that allows it to "perch" atop the neck. You might want to move the chair to a wall and place a pillow or cushion behind the head and neck so that your head can rest into that support behind you. Make yourself comfortable with a blanket, remove your glasses, and do anything else that would allow you to better relax for a few moments.

14. Close your eyes and scan your body from toes to head. Notice each set of joints you just warmed up. Observe any qualities of your skeleton as a whole. Does it feel stable or mobile, heavy or light, warm or cool? Do you notice anything about the soft tissue of your body—muscles, tendons, ligaments? Are they loose or tight? Energized or relaxed? Strong or soft? Notice your circulation, your nervous system, and the energy that moves

through your body. Observe any lines of communication that may have opened throughout the body from this movement.

15. *Pranayama*: Continue the theme of lubrication with a smooth breath. Begin by noticing the breath quality. At what stages of the breath are there stutters, pauses, or vibrations? When does the breath speed up or slow down? What feels easy and what requires more effort as you breathe? Begin to smooth the breath. If there are pauses, try to spread the breath across those gaps. If there are stutters or vibrations, pay close attention to calming and slowing the breath so it becomes more fluid. Certain phases of the breath will cooperate with this intention more readily than others. Simply continue to smooth each inhale, exhale, and transition between the two. Feel the breath open up spaces in the body for greater fluidity and ease. Practice for 30 seconds to five minutes then acknowledge the affect the smoother breath has on your sense of balance and contentment.

16. Release the focus on the breath and allow it to happen naturally and without concern. Let the mind rest, open and clear. Spend a few moments in ease and peace.

17. When you are ready, gently open the eyes. Notice your body and the space around you. Give a big stretch, waking up the body. Slowly begin to return to the happenings of your day, continuing to use these practices whenever feels right for you.

POSTURE, RELAXATION, BREATHING, CONCENTRATION: *VINYASA*: SUN SALUATION IN A CHAIR

This sequence is often used as a warm-up; however, it is safer for people with arthritis and similar conditions to warm up the body in other ways before performing this more intense sequence of backward and forward bending movements. The following practice takes the traditional Sun Salutation (*Surya Namaskar*) and adapts it so that the entire flow is performed seated in a chair. Images for this sequence are available in the Appendix:[130]

1. Seated Mountain: Sit forward in a firm chair, so that you are supporting your own spine. Knees should be in line with the hip joints and ankles directly under the knees. Shrug your shoulders to your ears and then allow the shoulder blades to gently slide down and rest on the back of the ribcage. Chin is parallel to the floor with the crown of head lengthening upward. Gaze is soft. Breathe fully and deeply.

2. Backbend (Inhale): Lengthen the arms forward or out to the sides and reach upward as high as feels comfortable for your shoulders. Open the heart and throat, lifting the sternum slightly without dropping the head backward.

3. Forward Fold (Exhale): Lengthen the spine and hinge forward at the hips, perhaps bringing the hands to the thighs, another chair, or a prop on the floor. Some people may be able to touch the floor.

4. Left Lunge (Inhale): Perch on the left side of the chair, holding onto the far edge of its seat with the right hand. Slide the left foot back so that the left knee lowers toward the floor. Keep the core engaged to support the low back. You might extend the left arm upward and arch slightly back, gazing up toward the hand. (If your chair has arms, you can do the lunge by sliding the left foot under the chair without turning 90 degrees.)

5. Downward Dog (Exhale): Turn back to center. Lengthen the spine and extend the arms alongside the ears or to whatever extent is available to you. Ground through the sitz bones on the chair and lengthen the fingertips away from the chair in opposition.

6. Cobra (Inhale): Place hands or elbows firmly on the thighs. Lengthen the spine and hinge forward, bending the elbows in close to the body. This should not be a forcing of the shoulder blades together and down—rather, a gentle gliding away from the ears and towards one another to open the chest and front of the shoulders. Lengthen through the crown of head and lift with the head, neck, and chest, looking out and up.

7. Downward dog (Exhale) as in Step 5 above.

8. Right Lunge (Inhale): Turn 90 degrees to the left, holding onto the chair with the left arm, and slide the right leg back in a lunge. Consider lifting the right arm and adding a slight backbend as in Step 4 above.

9. Forward Fold (Exhale): Return to center and fold forward as in Step 3, bending as far as feels comfortable.

10. Backbend (Inhale): Walk the hands up the legs to center and reach upward with a slight arch of the upper back.

11. Seated Mountain (Exhale): Bring the hands to the heart or your lap and return to relaxed breath.

12. Repeat on the other side.

13. You may move through this sequence a number of times. Notice how each repetition reveals changes in your strength, mobility, breath, emotions, and state of mind. You may also use this practice as a warm-up then continue on with some of the other sequences in this chapter.

14. *Pranayama*: Practice the Balanced Breath described in Chapter 2.

15. Following this Sun Salutation in a chair and *pranayama*, you may perform a visualization relaxation. Do any additional movement that feels appropriate to bring your body into balance and comfort before settling against the seatback. Maintain an upright and relaxed position, closing the eyes, and begin to imagine yourself in nature at dawn. Perhaps you are looking over the ocean or a lake; maybe you are on a tall hill or at a scenic lookout. Envision all the glorious colors of the sky and observe the deep sense of peace that is not only within you but all around, too. Perceive the sun peeking above the horizon, glowing pink and red. As you continue to relax, imagine all the changes in the sky, clouds, and sun as the day brightens. Imagine the warmth of the rising sun penetrating your whole being, soothing the heart, energizing the body, easing the mind. To transform this relaxation practice into a meditation, hold your mind on a still snapshot of dawn. The stillness and beauty harmonize with your thoughts and being. As you are ready, return to an awareness of this moment. Moving back into daily life, take the warmth and brightness of this image into your own day. Imagine yourself as a beacon of the sun's light and warmth in every encounter. Namaste.

POSTURE, CONCENTRATION: *VINYASA*: MOON SALUTATION (*CHANDRA NAMASKAR*)

This flowing sequence carries a quiet, introspective intention. It includes a lot of hip rotation and flexion, so if you have hip challenges, perform smaller movements and be mindful. For support, you may want to place a chair or two blocks on each side of the mat, which can reduce the intensity of some poses in the sequence. Although it requires strength, this can be a calming practice for the nervous system when performed slowly, taking multiple breaths in each posture before proceeding to the next. Each pose is a symbol for a phase of the moon, which reminds us to accept the ever-changing nature of life and the fluid nature of our emotions. This practice takes the body out of the typical forward-backward action we are accustomed to and provides lateral movements to increase mobility. Use it at the beginning or end of a practice or on its own as your *asana* practice that day. If you use this sequence as a warm-up, be sure to keep your movements at the minimum edge of sensation. If you are already warmed up, you may explore a deeper intensity as long as you are within the range of comfortable sensation. Remain mindful of the breath guiding the movement, keeping it deep, fluid and steady; in this way, the sequence becomes both an *asana* and a *pranayama* practice. You will want to stand with your mat running side to side, instead of the front-back orientation used in Sun Salutation:

1. Mountain Pose (*Tadasana*): Begin standing with feet hip (joint) distance apart, arms resting comfortably at your sides. Breathe deeply and feel connected, grounded, and calm.

2. Side-Bending Mountain (*Parsva Tadasana*): Reach your arms out to the sides and raise them as far overhead as feels comfortable. Keep the weight centered between both legs creating space in the hip joints. Without jutting the hip to either side, bend to the right from the waist. Return to center then side bend left. Come back to center.

3. Goddess Pose (*Deviasana*): Step the left foot further to the left side. Point the toes slightly outward in this wide-legged stance. Bend both knees, ensuring that they track over the ankles, not past them. Bring the arms into cactus position, with elbows bent to 90 degrees and fingers pointing upward (or however is comfortable). Feel strength in the upper legs and gluteal muscles.

4. Five-Pointed Star Pose (*Utthita Tadasana*): Straighten the knees to stand tall and wide. Straighten the elbows so the arms reach out, parallel to the floor. Gaze straight ahead.

5. Triangle Pose (*Trikonasana*): Turn the left foot to the left side, right foot turned in slightly, and shift the torso toward the left leg. Tilt sideways until the hand naturally reaches a place on the shin, block, or chair. Keep shoulder over shoulder, opening the right side of the body toward the ceiling without reaching so far that the spine begins to rotate. Gaze can be upward, straight ahead, or down toward the floor, depending on how this feels for your neck. Arms create one line from wrist to wrist, perpendicular to the floor, or place the right hand on the right hip.

6. Intense Side Stretch Pose (*Parsvottanasana*): For joint safety, return to an upright posture and straighten the legs before rotating the torso to the left. After turning to face the left leg, fold the torso forward, ensuring that the knee is not locked. The pelvis is squared to the left side, so that the right hip is reaching forward and the left hip is reaching back. Hands can be on the left leg, blocks, or chair.

7. Warrior I (*Virabhadrasana I*): Bend the left knee as your weight shifts forward over the left ankle (not past it). With hands on the chair, blocks, or left thigh, rise upright with a long spine. Bring arms overhead, hands to the hips, or wherever is comfortable.

8. Goddess Pose (*Deviasana*): Straighten the left leg and rotate back to center, turning the legs out from the hips so the toes point outward about 45 degrees. Bend the legs wide, knees over (not past) ankles, arms in cactus shape out to the sides.

9. Warrior I (*Virabhadrasana I*): Turn the right foot to the side, left foot pointing slightly right. Bend the right knee as your weight shifts forward over the right ankle. Lift the chest and face, mirroring the pose you did a few breaths ago. Place the arms wherever feels comfortable.

10. Intense Side Stretch Pose (*Parsvottanasana*): Begin to straighten the right leg and fold the torso toward it, so you repeat Step 5 on the other side. Right hip moves back and left hip moves forward, being sure not to lock the front knee.

11. Triangle Pose (*Trikonasana*): Come up to standing and rotate the torso forward, then reach the torso right coming into Triangle on the right side. Hand may lower to the chair, block, or right leg. Torso turns upward opening the left side body with neck in a comfortable orientation. Left arm may reach upward or left hand may rest on the left hip.

12. 5-Pointed Star Pose (*Utthita Tadasana*): Straighten out of Triangle Pose. Turn the legs outward from the hips and reach the arms out to the sides.

13. Goddess Pose (*Deviasana*): Bend the knees to the sides, ensuring that they track over the ankles. Bend the elbows, as the hands point upwards.

14. Side-bending Mountain (*Parsva Tadasana*): Reach your arms out to the sides and raise them as far overhead as feels right. Bring legs back to center, keeping hips square. Lengthen the spine upward and bend to the left from the waist. Return to center then repeat on the other side.

15. Mountain Pose (*Tadasana*): Lower the arms and feel the effects of this sequence on body, mind, and spirit. You may repeat this sequence, stepping out to the right this time. When you have completed the Moon Salutations, pause and experience a sense of grounded fluidity.

16. Moon Meditation: Stand or sit comfortably on a chair or the floor and call to mind an image of the moon. Perhaps you wish to focus on the dark, quiet potential of a new moon, the growth or recession of a half-moon, or the bright realization of a full moon. On different days you may want to call upon different moon phases. Hold in your mind the image of a peaceful night sky and the presence of the moon. You may sense how the moon pulls the waters of your body, just as it pulls the tides. You may allow your consciousness to become absorbed by the image or feeling of the moon. If your mind wanders, just bring it back to that lunar focus. After five or ten minutes, carry the sense of peacefulness with you as you return to your day.

POSTURE, RELAXATION: RESTORATIVE SEQUENCE

Restorative poses allow the body to truly let go. As you move through the following sequence, encourage your body to release and rely on the support beneath it. You can think of this action as a metaphor for life. Are there places in life where you can sink into the support that is available to you? Are there friends and family whose support you resist? Community resources you haven't accessed? Assistive devices you could utilize more frequently? Throughout this restorative sequence, notice how you are able to sink into postures, and also notice when you resist letting go. This may provide some insight into other areas of your life. You may want to perform these poses in bed, using your blankets and pillows as props. Stay in each pose for five to ten minutes, giving yourself ample time to genuinely drop into it. If time is a limiting factor, you may select just one posture and perform it for an extended period.

While dedicated breathing practices often happen at the beginning or end of a yoga class, the breath should continue to be mindfully engaged throughout any yoga practice. As we are mindful of the breath throughout movement practice, we are practicing a form of *pranayama* all along. For restorative practice, begin prolonging the exhale. This *rechaka pranayama* engages the parasympathetic (relaxation) response. Let the inhale take care of itself and focus on elongating the exhale. You may notice various thoughts and emotions pass; simply breathe them away on that long out-breath. In this way, the mind is supported by the breath just as the body is supported by the props:

1. Forward Bend (Figure 11.1): If you can comfortably come to the floor, sit down facing a chair with pillows and/or blankets handy. You may want to sit up on some cushions in order to avoid discomfort in the low back. You can widen your legs so that they extend on either side of the chair and you may need a rolled towel under your knees for support. Lean forward so that your forehead rests on the chair. You might rest your forehead on the back of your hands or place a cushion on the chair for softness. You can also do this sitting in a chair with the forehead resting on a pillow against the wall. The intentional attitude (bhavana) of a forward fold is to surrender, to be grounded without effort. You can try any other variations on a forward bend, but this should not be a stretching pose. It is a pose for

letting go. Use the props to play around and support any parts of the body that need it. Allow yourself to melt into that support.

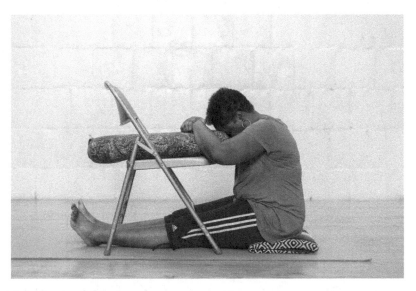

Figure 11.1: Forward Bend

2. Side Bend (Figure 11.2): This can be easily done lying in bed. The idea is to have a slight lateral curve in the spine to energetically open the side body. Lying on one side, you may want to have a pillow between the knees so that the thighs can be parallel to each other. Place a pillow underneath your head so that the neck is properly aligned. In this position, you also want to place a pillow or blanket under the ribcage. This will allow for a slight side-bending position. Again, it should not feel like a big stretch and you should be able to let the body relax into this support. You may have the upper arm overhead alongside the ear or resting on a cushion in front of you. After a few minutes, roll to the other side to repeat the posture there. You may notice that the two sides feel differently and that you need slightly different support on the second side. We are all asymmetrical, so see if you can notice and respond to that difference with curiosity, not concern. Enjoy breathing into the open side of your body.

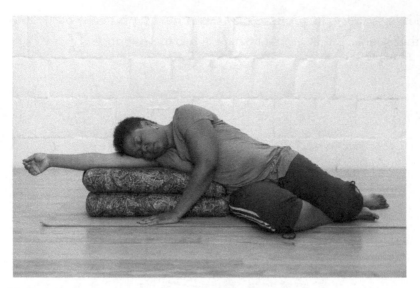

Figure 11.2: Side Bend

3. Back Bend (Figure 11.3): This pose will be done lying on your back, either on the floor or bed. You will probably want a pillow or other support under the knees to alleviate any pressure on the low back. Additionally, place a pillow or other support under the back, from the hips to the armpits. If this is not comfortable, you might try rolling a large towel and placing it directly along the spine from tailbone to head. In either scenario, you should feel an opening in the chest, heart, and front of the torso. Notice the space this creates for the inhale, as you continue to prolong the exhale. You may want to be covered with a blanket to feel protected and secure. Be sure to support any parts of the body that need it. If a restorative pose is not comfortable, you just haven't found the right variation yet. It can take some playing around, but when you find it, you should feel ease in the body and the ability to let go.

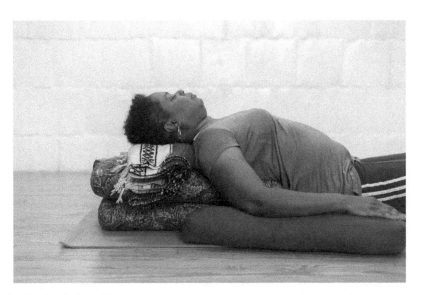

Figure 11.3: Back Bend

4. Twist (Figure 11.4): Remove the props from under the body so that you are lying on your back with a pillow or other support on your left side. Draw the right knee in toward the chest and then let it fall across the body to rest on the left pillow. You can bring some support under the right shoulder, which may have lifted off the floor. Consider any other parts of the body that are not able to fully relax and put a blanket, cushion, or block beneath them. You may even want more support under the right leg. This should feel like a gentle twist through the whole spine. After a few minutes, roll onto the back and rock side to side a few times before moving into the posture on the other side.

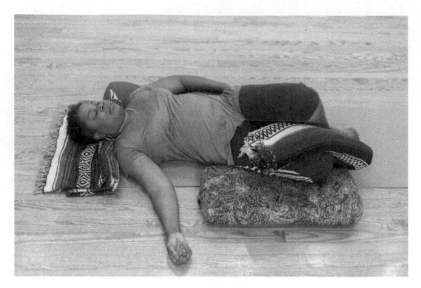

Figure 11.4: Twist

5. Supported *Savasana* (Figure 11.5): Remain lying on your back with a cushion beneath the knees, taking pressure off the lower back. You may also want a small rolled towel beneath the natural curve in neck. You may add some other form of weight that helps you feel more present, supported, or grounded, such as a blanket over the whole body, a cushion on the torso, or props over the upturned palms of the hands. Feel all the points of connection and allow that feeling to deepen as you rest and release down. Remain in this posture and focus on the surface beneath you. Feel the resistance as you inhale, inflating the lungs and creating pressure against the bed or floor. Feel the release as you exhale. Allow each out breath to be a little longer than the last as you continue to release and relax. When you are ready to come out of the posture, gently roll on your side then use your hands and arms to help you return to a seated position, carrying the sense of being supported with you. Take a few breaths to acknowledge the relaxation and freedom the practice created.

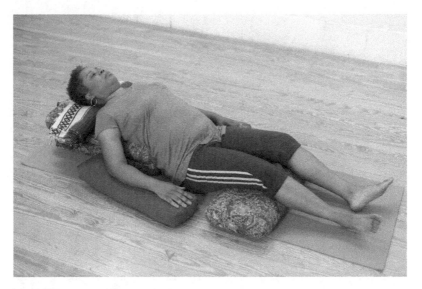

Figure 11.5: Supported Savasana

These restorative postures are useful any time you feel worn out. They can be practiced in bed to ease yourself into your day or help bring sleep at night. If you don't have much time, it is okay to rest in just one or two of these postures and bask in a place of ease.

Summary

This chapter highlighted the fundamentals of sequencing a home yoga practice and offered a few basic sequences. As you grow more comfortable with the routines and your individual responses to yoga, feel free to experiment with and adapt movements in the context of your own comfort and safety. If you are attending yoga classes, rehabilitation, or yoga therapy, consider incorporating some of those movements and postures as well. Diversifying your practice can keep you engaged and bring new perspective to a common routine. The next chapter gives you more sequences you can experiment with and apply to help you or your clients cope with arthritis.

Chapter 12

SEQUENCES FOR SPECIFIC INTENTIONS

Building on the pose adaptations, warm-up sequences, and home practice structure provided in the previous chapter, this chapter includes additional practices and short sequences. I have learned in my own life and through my work with clients that the commitment to an hour-long daily home practice is not always sustainable for a variety of reasons. I find that incorporating smaller practices throughout the day infuses life with the fundamental concepts of yoga when they are most needed. Feel free to use these shorter sequences on their own, or combine them in whatever way seems interesting or useful. Please remember that the Appendix contains many pose variations, so use those to find more comfort and ease in the practice. Don't feel limited by the variations I offer, because the options are really limitless. Explore ways of being in each pose with a sense of curiosity and see what else you might find. As you do so, consider the guidelines in the previous chapter to optimize safety and ground the practice in *ahimsa* (non-harm).

POSTURE, RELAXATION, BREATHING, CONCENTRATION: YOGA PRACTICE SUPPORTED BY A CHAIR

This practice uses the chair for support without actually sitting in it. Make sure all four feet of the chair are on the sticky mat at all times to prevent slipping. This sequence also requires you to have a second sticky mat crossing the first, to make a plus sign on the floor. (Alternatively, you can turn your body back and forth as needed, using only one mat.) Play with how much you use the chair or play with letting go for moments or longer. Have fun!

Perform one of the warming up practices recommended in this or the previous chapter, perhaps beginning with joint movements and then Sun/Moon Salutations:

1. Mountain Pose (*Tadasana*): Find a steady, strong Mountain Pose. Feet are hip joint distance apart and dropping into the support of the floor. Knees are soft, not locked. Tailbone melts downward without tucking to create space in the low back. The core is engaged and allows the movement of full deep breath. Shoulders soften back and down while the spine lengthens. Head floats gently on the spine. The gaze is relaxed, as is the mind.

2. Eagle Pose (*Garudasana*): Start by gradually shifting weight from one side to the other and notice how the whole body shifts slightly as you bring more weight into one foot and then the other. Settle onto your right foot, holding the back of the chair for balance. Create length in the supporting leg, so that you find space in the hip and are not sinking into it. Bring the left leg in front of the right, crossing at the thigh, knee, or shin. See what happens when you bend the knees and hips deeply, reaching the tailbone back. You might want to place the left foot or ankle on a block to the left of your right foot. Try placing right hand on left shoulder or, if you are stable without holding the chair, bring the arms straight in front of you. Either hug your torso or cross at the forearms or elbows, keeping the energy of the heart open and the length in the spine. Some people will bring back of hands or palms together, as long as fingertips still point upward, not in or down. Hands are positioned between the eyes. Notice the opposing twists. The lower body twists and crosses in one direction, while the upper body twists and crosses in the other direction, bringing the body back to

center. Be mindful of joint discomfort and adjust accordingly. Find a point in front of you at eye height and fix your visual attention for a few breaths. Unwind with awareness. Find *Tadasana* again and notice the difference between right and left side before repeating on the other side.

3. Warrior III Pose (*Virabhadrasana III*): Step back slightly from the chair, holding onto its back for safety and support. Keeping length in the spine, hinge forward at the hips, raising the left leg behind you. Imagine a long line of energy from the left foot to the crown of the head as you reach back through the left heel. The head stays aligned with the spine, so your gaze will lower as you move. Tip only as far forward as feels stable, keeping a tiny bend in the right knee so it doesn't lock. Keep the weight of the body distributed through the whole sole of the foot, so that you aren't leaning back into the right heel. You might only tilt 10–15 degrees, or you might extend 90 degrees until the body is parallel to the floor. This will depend on your stability and flexibility in the pose. Feel free to extend the right arm overhead or hold the chair, or put it into a cactus position, or out to the side. Inhale to lengthen and exhale to slowly lower out of the pose, finding *Tadasana*. Pause and observe, then repeat on the other side.

4. Warrior II Pose (*Virabhadrasana II*): Step wide on your mat, holding the arms straight out to the sides, with wrists and shoulders in one line (or wrists below shoulders if that feels better). Think about stepping so wide that your feet are under your palms, or as wide as feels comfortable for you. You may hold the back of the chair or sit on the edge of the seat so that most of your body weight is supported by the chair. The right leg rotates 90 degrees so that the toes point directly outward. The left leg rotates inward so that the toes of the back foot angle in 45 degrees. You might want a wedge or other support under that back foot. Hips remain squared with the shoulders. Gaze turns over the right shoulder, being sure not to lower the left arm as you do so. Watch the alignment of the knee as it tracks over the ankle. If necessary, widen the stance so you can bend deeper without the knee extending beyond the ankle. Balance the weight evenly through right and left ball of the foot and heel, like a tripod, so the weight is not rolling to the inside or outside of the foot. Gaze out past the right arm. Shoulders relax away from the ears and the fingertips are lengthened with energy reaching out to both sides. Feel the intense focus

of Warrior energy in this pose. From here, proceed to Reverse Warrior then repeat them both on the other side.

5. Reverse Warrior Pose: From the Warrior II stance, turn the right palm upward. Leaning the torso back, the left hand comes to rest on the outside of the left leg. It is not important how far down the leg it reaches as it simply rests there for stability. If you are comfortable releasing your hold of the chair, the right (front) arm can reach overhead in an arc, with the gaze up at the right hand. Adjust the position of the arm and head for the comfort of your shoulders and neck. Feel an opening in the whole right side body. Return to center, straighten the right knee, and walk the feet in for *Tadasana* before moving into Warrior II on the other side.

6. Side Angle Pose (*Utthita Parsvakonasana*): Return to the Warrior II stance with the right knee bent and lean right, holding the chair back with the right hand or bringing the right elbow to rest on the right thigh. You may also perform this perched on the chair seat. Feel a line of energy reaching from the back left foot and out the crown of the head. You can extend the left arm alongside the left ear to give a complete stretch through the left side of the body, or place the left hand on the left hip. Your gaze might be past the extended fingers or straight forward. Avoid leaning too heavily into the chair or supporting elbow; instead, keep neck long and shoulders square and strong, in one plane, as though laying against a wall. Feel energy through the upper side of the body. After a few breaths, inhale back to center and repeat on the other side or move into the next pose before repeating both on the other side.

7. Half-Moon Pose (*Ardha Chandrasana*): The chair should be to your right side. Standing in Side Angle Pose or coming back into a Warrior II stance, shift your weight into the right leg, so that you are able to come up onto the left toes. The left leg may naturally slide in closer to the right leg as you reach for the seat of the chair with your right hand. The palm, fist, or fingertips can rest on the chair seat. When you feel secure with your connection to the chair, begin lifting the left leg off of the floor, only as much as feels accessible and safe. You might even want to try this pose against the wall the first few times for stability and safety. Stand close to the back of the chair, holding it for support. Strengthen the muscles through the back of the leg and lower back, engaging them to inhale and

lift the right leg behind you. Think about stacking the left shoulder over the right shoulder, feeling an opening in the left side of the torso. You may want to bring the left hand to the left hip or reach it up toward the ceiling. Gaze forward or upward, whichever feels better for you. Be sure to continue breathing fully and deeply throughout the experience of the pose. The fullness of the breath supports balance and helps to reduce tension in the body during challenging poses. As you are ready, slowly lower the left foot back into Warrior II position and bring the torso upright. Return to *Tadasana* to repeat on the other side, being sure that there is a chair available to support you.

8. Wide-Legged Forward Fold (*Prasarita Padottanasana*): Face the seat of the chair, standing about a foot away. Step wide, as if preparing for Warrior II. Be sure that neither you nor the chair can slip. Hinge forward from the hip joint and bring hands, fists, or elbows to the seat of the chair or to blocks set on the seat. Keep the spine long and ensure the sensation is in the thick part of your hamstrings, not behind the knees or around the hips. Let yourself adjust the angle of your feet, bend in your knees, support of the chair, and whatever else you may need to shift for comfort in the pose. Find surrender, release, and respite from the day. Allow your exhale to lengthen as you begin to unwind from the previous challenges of this sequence. As you are ready, step the feet in more narrowly to come up. Bring hands to the thighs with knees bent and keep a long spine as you press up to vertical. If you get a head rush, hold the chair with one hand and raise the other overhead to equalize blood pressure as you take a deep breath.

9. Legs Up a Chair Pose: Use the chair for support in getting down to the floor (in reverse order to what is described in Chapter 2 on getting up from the floor). Lie down with your hips close to the chair seat, knees bent and feet flat on the floor. You may want a folded blanket or pillow under the sacrum, along the spine, or rolled under the neck. Bring the lower legs up onto the chair, so both calves are supported by the chair while the rest of the body lies comfortably on the floor. Depending on bone length, you may need to adjust the position of the chair or your body so that the thighs are perpendicular to the floor, knees lined up over the hip joints. Hands can rest on belly, chest, or extend out to the sides as in *Savasana*. In this

position, let the weight of the body release into its support. You may want to close the eyes and notice the natural deepening of the breath.

10. Releasing Breath: Breathe in deeply. When you exhale, do so with an audible sigh, such as, "Ahhhh…" As you repeat this a few times, play with how long you make each out breath, and the kinds of sounds you make. Be playful and also listen to yourself. Relax as you allow yourself to let go of held stresses, frustrations, and beliefs with the sound and energy of your sighs.

11. Relaxation: Allow your breath to find its own deep, regular place as it balances your nervous system. As your mind unwinds, you let go of thoughts about whatever transpired during the practice. Release what has passed and what is to come. Exhale by exhale, bring your awareness back to the breath relaxing the body and mind.

12. Meditation: After a few minutes of relaxation, bring the legs off of the chair, and roll onto one side in a fetal position. Use the arms to support you as you come to sitting, perhaps on a prop or on the chair. Focus on an uplifting idea, perhaps one that arose from practice, by creating a short mantra, word, sound, image, or feeling that represents it. Bask in the meaning of that focus. When your mind wanders, as is its nature, simply bring it back to the focus you chose. When it is time to come out of the meditation, acknowledge the effects of practice on your sense of wellbeing, emotions, thoughts, breath, and body. Through the rest of your day, you may want to invoke the practice by recalling your focus or simply heaving a pleasant sigh.

POSTURE, RELAXATION, BREATHING: PREVENTING AND MANAGING KNEE ARTHRITIS

This sequence is beneficial for people with many different forms of arthritis. Those with OA are commonly affected in the knees. Those with larger bodies may also find this to be an important practice:

1. Begin seated in a chair. You may place folded blankets or extra cushions under the seat for support or for longer limbs. If your feet do not reach the floor, place them on blocks or another elevating prop. Keep the ankles aligned beneath the knees, which are also in line with the hip joints so that the femur (thigh bone) is parallel to the floor. Close the eyes to help focus on breath awareness, gradually increasing diaphragmatic or Three-Part Breath (see Chapter 3) to activate the parasympathetic response. Let go of whatever may have happened before the present moment, or what is yet to be. Be with your breath, emotions, and thoughts as they are now.

2. Seated Mountain Pose (*Tadasana*): Sit tall and imagine the expansion of your intervertebral discs as you lengthen and create space. Keep the chin parallel to the floor and soften the muscles of the face as you breathe deeply. Send energy out the fingertips as the arms lengthen down toward the floor in opposition to the lengthening spine.

3. Brief Warm-Up of Joint Articulations, as described in the previous chapter.

4. One-Leg Lift: Ensure that the knees are a hip width apart. Sitting up tall, hold onto the sides of the chair. Inhale as you straighten one knee to raise the lower leg. Press out through the heel. It's okay if your leg doesn't straighten all the way or if the muscles shake as they gain strength. Exhale and slowly lower the leg down. Acknowledge the strength you are building through the thighs and stabilizers around the knee joint. Repeat this practice on the other side, continuing to link breath and movement.

5. Side Bend: Carry on with the movements of Step 5 as you add a side stretch. Inhale to raise the left leg, keeping a nice long spine and hands holding the chair. With the leg extended, reach the left arm overhead as high as feels comfortable (if you feel stable doing so), exhale and side bend to the right. Feel the left torso and hip open as the right side strengthens. Inhale the torso to center then lower the arm and exhale the leg down. Repeat on the other side.

6. Seated Staff Pose (*Dandasana*): This movement requires more core support and strength. Slide all the way back in the chair so that the chair back is supporting you. Hold the sides of the chair and inhale to straighten both knees. If you round in the low back (rolling back on the pelvis), it is a sign to return to one-legged lifts instead. Even if your feet do not lift off

the floor, the attempt at this posture engages the muscles that can improve stability. Be sure you continue to sit up tall and allow the back of the chair to support you.

7. Seated Balance: As you perform Seated Staff Pose, consider raising one arm overhead. Notice how the muscles throughout your body work to hold you stable. Lower arm and legs for a few breaths and then raise the legs again, this time lifting the other arm. For a greater challenge, you might try raising both arms with the legs extended. Send your breath anywhere you feel tension and holding, such as the shoulders, jaw, or eyes. Notice the difference between strength and tension.

8. Wide-Angle Forward Bend (*Upavistha Konasana*): Keep your sitz bones back in the chair and take the legs wider apart, feet still on blocks if appropriate, with the knees over the ankles. Hinge at the hips to lengthen the spine towards the top of the thighs. You may support with hands or elbows on knees or hands/fingertips/fists on tall blocks alongside the legs or between them. You can also place your hands on the seat of another chair in front of you.

9. Forward-Folding Twist (*Parivritta Janu Sirsasana*): Maintaining the fold, begin to bring the right shoulder towards the floor. Repeat on the other side. You can bring hands to knees for support. You may move with the breath, exhaling to twist and inhaling to center, or hold the twist for a few breaths on each side. Come back to center with a long spine and, using the hands for support, inhale to sit tall.

10. Seated Pigeon (*Eka Pada Kapotasana*): Cross the right ankle over the left knee or place the right foot/ankle on a tall block to the outside of the left foot. Exhale and hinge the hips to angle the torso forward, keeping a long spine. Note you may not need to angle forward in order to feel the stretch in the iliotibial band and outside of the right thigh. Find a position where you feel a gentle stretch without pulling or forcing. A flexed right foot increases the intensity of the stretch and helps protect the knee. Repeat on the other side.

11. Chair Pose (*Utkatasana*): While still seated in the chair with feet firmly planted on the floor, imagine what happens in the body as you prepare to stand. This posture strengthens the muscles of independence, the

quadriceps in the thighs, which help bring you from sitting to standing. Without rising, engage the muscles that help you get from seated to standing. Relax. Take a deep breath in, and on the exhale, engage those muscles again, leaning slightly forward, pressing the palms to the thighs for support, and raise the hips an inch from the chair. Lower back to the chair and relax. Inhale, and on the exhale press into the feet, engage the thigh muscles, and rise again. This time, bring the weight more firmly into the feet to breathe steadily as you hold yourself up before exhaling and relaxing down. You may guide yourself up and down by holding the sides of the chair. When you hold the posture, ensure that your weight is evenly distributed through the heels and balls of the feet. Imagine right angles at the knees and hips. You may move through this lift and lower sequence a few times, guided by the breath. Finally, inhale and using the hands on the thighs for support with a nice long spine, press yourself through Chair Pose all the way to standing. You may want to take a few breaths in Mountain or shake out the arms and legs before returning to the chair. Use your hands to support and guide as necessary as you move back to being seated again. Getting up from a chair safely and independently is an important life skill for those who do not use assistive devices such as a walker or wheelchair. If you do not have the mobility or strength to rise from the chair, engaging those muscles in preparation may help to slowly build the capacity to execute this movement.

12. Seated Warrior I with Side Bend: Slide over to the left side of the chair and slide the left leg out behind you while your right hand holds the right side of the chair seat. Inhale the left arm up and exhale to side bend right. You may look toward the chair, floor, or up to the ceiling instead. Bring the leg back to the starting position, move to the left side of the chair and repeat on the other side. This can also be done by rotating in the chair to the right, holding the chair back with the right hand, sliding the left leg behind and stretching to the right. Either way, the left toes can be relaxed on the floor or turned under while the right foot is firmly planted with a 90-degree angle at the knee. This is an opportunity to stretch the hip flexor muscles that are flexed while sitting.

13. Seated Twist Pose (*Ardha Matsyendrasana*): Turn right to face sideways in the chair, with both feet on the floor. Sit tall and twist slowly to the right,

holding onto the back of the chair without pulling or forcing, just allowing a gentle twist through the whole spine. You can check your position by raising the hands. If your body does not change position, you know that you are not over-using the arms. This also highlights the core muscles needed to maintain a healthy, upright twist. Release to center, pausing there and observing the difference between right and left side as you notice the effects of the twist. Exhale, twist to the right again. You may raise the hands to check yourself, breathing normally as you hold the twist or make this posture dynamic by exhaling into the twist and inhaling back to center. After you have repeated the twist a few times, face the left side and twist to the left. Be sure to perform the posture with the same method and duration as you did on the right.

14. Seated Corpse Pose (*Savasana*): Bring the chair against the wall, support the neck with a cushion and rest the head against the wall. Prop your limbs and torso however you need to so that this posture feels effortless. You might want a pillow on your lap to rest the arms, a folded blanket on the feet to feel grounded, or a blanket covering your whole body for coziness. Consider dimming the lights as you bring your awareness inward.

15. Grounded Relaxation: Feel yourself drop into the support of the chair, wall, and floor. Let go of any tension, holding, or effort. Imagine your feet growing roots into the earth. Allow that relaxation to move into the ankles, calves, shins. The relaxation travels into the knees. Feel an opening in the joint: spacious, cool, calm knees. Feel relaxation in the thighs, allowing them to let go after putting forth effort. The relaxation travels up into the hip joints. Feel the weight of the pelvis dropping into the chair. Relaxation moves from the hips and pelvis up into the low back, middle back, and upper back. Imagine space between all the vertebrae of the spine, relaxing all the muscles of the back, chest, and belly so the whole torso is long and relaxed. Let the tips of the fingers soften and feel that relaxation move into the palms, back of the hands and wrists. Soften the forearms, elbows, and upper arms. Shoulder joints are open and calm; the jaw slackens, teeth unclenched, tongue relaxed in the mouth. Feel the eyes soften in their sockets, the tiny muscles relaxing through the face, hairline, over the skull. Allow the breath to deepen. Each exhale allows you to let go of anything not serving you in this moment as you relax more deeply.

Although thoughts may be moving through the mind, you allow them to pass without concern, staying relaxed in body, breath, and mind. Enjoy a few minutes of calm and quiet. When you are ready, begin to move gently, perhaps wiggling the fingers and toes or turning the head side to side. Bring yourself away from the wall so that you are sitting tall and supporting your own spine in a seated *Tadasana*.

16. Cooling Breath (*Sheetali Pranayama*): Once you have returned to a tall, upright position, begin to practice the cooling breath outlined in Chapter 7. Feel the cool air bringing a sense of calm to the body and mind with each breath. After a few minutes of this practice, pause and acknowledge its effects on all levels of your person, including your overall sense of wellbeing.

This sequence brings strength to the muscles that stabilize the knees, mobility to the soft tissues, and cooling sensations to an inflamed system. It is accessible to a variety of levels of experience, practice, and health. It is recommended as an everyday practice and can be adapted for greater challenge or gentleness, depending upon your current needs. The following practice builds greater strength through standing poses, using the wall or a chair for support.

POSTURE, RELAXATION, BREATHING: MINI-SEQUENCE: FINDING STEADINESS IN UNCERTAINTY

Arthritis is an unpredictable disease. On any given day, we cannot predict what pain levels will be, the degree of fatigue or what other physical, mental, or social concerns may impact contentment, comfort, and peace of mind. The uncertainty of arthritis lies on top of the usual volatility of life. One never knows what may come, and this can be a source of great anxiety for some people. The following practice recruits physical stability to offer you a sense of steadiness in the face of uncertainty. Remember to seek mental health support for your anxiety and supplement it with yoga. While this practice is not a clinical treatment for anxiety, it is a beneficial practice for combating its symptoms and to re-center yourself when life seems unpredictable or out of control. Practice the first two steps every time. Beyond that, you can mix and match any of the remaining steps as time and energy allows:

1. Settle into Mountain Pose, equalizing your weight on the tripod of each foot; quads and core are active and relaxed; the spine is long with a natural curve. Close your eyes (holding onto a chair for support as needed) and notice any rocking or movement you may perceive through your body. Allow the body to become more steady and still, noticing the role of breath, emotions, and thoughts in that process.

2. Warm up with small, slow movements of the head—front and back, side to side, left and right. Roll the shoulders and hips in both directions. Shake out the arms and legs, move the elbows and knees, roll out the wrists and ankles, wiggle the fingers and toes. After fully engaging and warming the body, let the movement settle. For a moment, return to Mountain Pose, close the eyes and steady yourself again.

3. Tree Pose (*Vrkasana*): You may want to try this pose with fingertips on the wall or a chair for stability. Begin by shifting your weight from right to left sides and notice how your torso moves as the weight distribution changes. Shift over to the left side so that the left foot is holding most of your weight, while lifting up through the torso to avoid sinking into the left hip. Imagine creating space in the left hip joint. Visualize your left foot growing roots through the floor, creating freedom on the right side. From that rootedness, rotate the right hip open with the right heel off the floor. You might try sliding the right foot up the inside of the left leg to increase the balance challenge, letting the foot remain anywhere above or below the knee. Avoid pressing the foot into the knee as this compromises the safety of the knee joint. Play with balance by experimenting with arm positions: hands on hips, cactus arms, arms to the side, behind, or overhead, or what variation you choose. Don't worry about symmetry if your shoulders do not have the same range of motion. Do whatever is comfortable for your joints and feels best for you. Notice the slight adaptations your body makes to keep you steady as your arms move. You might think of this as a metaphor for daily life; in order to be balanced in life, we are constantly adapting and adjusting to the moment as it changes. Lower the right foot back to the floor, pause in Mountain Pose and steady yourself. Repeat on the other side.

4. Warrior Pose I (*Virabhadrasana I*): From Mountain Pose, step the left foot back a comfortable distance. You may place a yoga wedge or other prop under the heel to ensure groundedness through the entire foot or turn the toes out to the side slightly (approximately 45 degrees) so that you can ground through the outside edge of the foot. Bend the right knee, ensuring that it doesn't extend past the right ankle. You might need to increase the length of your stance to make room for a deeper knee bend. To gain more stability, you can also try stepping the feet laterally wider apart. Hands can come to hips, overhead, or use one of your favorite arm variations. Keep the spine tall with shoulders back over the hips, core strong with space between ribs and hips, and gaze forward and focused but without strain. Imagine yourself as a hero midstride in a run, connecting to the strength and engagement in your front (right) leg and breathing rhythmically. You are facing whatever is in front of you with readiness and purpose. After a few breaths, step the back foot forward and the right foot back to repeat on the other side. Finish in a steadying Mountain Pose.

5. Half-Moon Pose (*Ardha Chandrasana*): Bring your sticky mat up to the wall so the long side of the mat is against the wall. Taller individuals might want a long mat or two mats end-to-end. Set one chair at each end with enough room between them for you to step wide. Rotate out at the hip to turn your right foot towards the front chair, holding onto it for support. Keep the knee unlocked and the quadriceps strong as you shift into the right foot and place your left foot on the seat of the other chair. Use the wall behind you for support, leaning on it with shoulders and/or hips. Experiment with how much you contact the wall. If you feel confident, you might want to leave a hair of space and endeavour to hold yourself steady, knowing the wall is close enough to catch you. Your right hand is still on the chair and your left hand can come to hip, shoulder, or overhead. Look down, straight ahead, or up—whichever is most comfortable for your neck. Bask in the expansiveness of this pose with limbs stretched out in all directions. When you are ready, come out of the pose by rotating the torso toward the ground, gripping the front chair with both hands, and lowering the left leg. Stand in Mountain pose to still yourself, then repeat on the other side.

6. *Pranayama*: Remain in a strong, steady Mountain Pose with eyes open or closed. Begin to balance the breath by equalizing the length of each inhale

and exhale. When the equal breath feels steady, lengthen it by adding a count to the inhale and then the exhale. Every few breaths, see if you can prolong it a little bit more. Notice the effects of this full, even breathing on mind, body, energy, and emotions.

7. Relaxation: Remain in Mountain Pose with your feet hip-width apart, placing both hands on the back of a chair for stability. Perform a body scan relaxation starting with the head and moving sequentially down until you have relaxed every part of you, all the way to the feet. Remain grounded as you go through your day, acknowledging your ability to bring yourself back to a steady center whenever it is needed.

POSTURE: MINI-SEQUENCE: DESK YOGA POSES

This sequence offers simple movements you can use while seated at a desk. This is a healthy way to nurture the body during long periods of desk work. The entire sequence of postures is performed seated in a chair:

1. Seated Mountain: Sit forward in a firm chair, so that you are supporting your own spine with your core muscles. Knees should be in line with the hip joints and ankles directly under the knees. Shoulders are back and down with a lengthened spine. Chin is parallel to the floor with the crown of head lengthening upward. Gaze is soft. Breathe fully and deeply. This pose can be a nice reminder to maintain healthy alignment throughout the day and to fully engage the breath.

2. Side Stretch: Starting in Mountain, hold onto the seat or arm of the chair with the left hand. Reach the right arm overhead, to cactus, or place the fingertips on the right shoulder. Inhale and lengthen through the spine from tailbone to crown of head. Use the left arm for support as you exhale, bending to the left, bringing the left ribs toward the left hip. Breathing deeply, keep both sitz bones grounded and feet firmly planted. On an inhale, return to center and repeat on the other side. This is a nice stretch for reducing compression in the spine.

3. Chair Warrior: Starting in Seated Mountain, turn 90 degrees in your chair to face the right. Slide back so that much of your thighs are supported by the chair. Open the left leg 90 degrees so that the left foot is on the floor to your left, with knee and ankle aligned. Lengthen the spine and twist to the left so that your torso is facing the same direction as your left knee. Take the arms out to the sides or to your hips or shoulders. You can also try extending the left leg and opening it as far to the left as feels available to you. Gaze over the right shoulder or out past the right fingertips. Experience the stability and intensity of this pose for a few breaths and then turn in your chair to find the same pose on the other side. This pose may help to foster inner strength, resolve, and focus.

4. Cat-Cow: Start in Mountain. Begin on an exhale by drawing the belly in as you reach the mid-back toward the chair back behind you. Roll onto the back of the sitz bones, lowering the head and rounding the upper back to create a C-curve in the spine. Return to center and inhale as you arch backwards to open the front of the body. Imagine the shoulder blades as two hands on the back ribs, with the bottom of the shoulder blades like the heels of the hands pressing forward and lifting the heart space. Reach the solar plexus forward. You might move through this sequence several times, exhaling as you round, inhaling as you arch the back. You might also find that it feels good to slide the hands along the thighs with each movement, so that they move toward the knees as you round forward and toward the hips as you arch backward. This pose helps to reduce stiffness in the spine and tension in the back muscles.

5. Seated Staff: Slide to the back of your chair so that you are supported by the chair back. Hold onto the sides of the chair or chair arms. Extend both legs forward, flexing the feet to bring your toes toward the ceiling, as if you were standing on a wall in front of you. Engage the thigh muscles and breathe deeply with a long spine, active neutral core and relaxed shoulders. After a few breaths, slowly return the feet to the floor and slide forward in your chair. This pose helps to build strength, stabilize the knees, and energize the body. It can also be done with one leg at a time to gradually build strength and stability.

6. Camel (*Ustrasana*): Stay sitting back in your chair so that you feel the top of the chair back making contact with your mid to upper back. Open the chest

and arch back, supported by the chair back. You can hold onto the chair seat, reach the arms behind you with the fingers pointing down toward the floor, or rest your arms on the arms of the chair. Open the heart and throat, lift the gaze slightly upward (without dropping the head back), and breathe deeply in this supported backbend for a few moments. Feel the opening in the whole front body and more fullness in the breath. After a few breaths, return to Seated Mountain and notice the changes on your seated posture. This pose can be useful for those who tend to sit forward or round over a keyboard or other device.

7. Seated Spinal Twist: Come forward on your chair to Seated Mountain. Keep the alignment of the hips, knees, and ankles and lengthen through the whole spine with shoulders relaxing down and in toward the spine. Gently begin to twist right, starting at the base of the spine and working upward one vertebrae at a time until finally the head turns to look over the right shoulder. You might want to bring the left hand to the right knee and the right hand to the chair seat or arm. Be sure not to pull or force the twist, just allow the movement that is possible naturally through the spine, ribs, and back. After a few breaths, return to center, roll the shoulders, lengthen the spine again, and slowly twist to the other side. Twists can help to improve the alignment of the spine in relationship to the shoulders and pelvis.

8. Return to Seated Mountain, softly gazing straight ahead. Inhale, reach both arms up alongside the ears, feeling yourself stretch out the top of the head, too. Exhale, lower the arms, and return to your deskwork feeling rejuvenated.

POSTURE: MINI-SEQUENCE: CULTIVATING INNER STRENGTH

Self-care requires personal strength and discipline (*tapas*). Some days we may feel too tired to prepare healthy meals, clean the house, connect with loved ones, fulfill work responsibilities, perform self-massage, and all the other major and minor details of healthy living. The following brief session of postures helps fortify the attitude and embodied experience of inner strength. Note that, although it is written as a standing practice, it can be readily adapted for a chair (see Appendix):

1. Stand in Mountain Pose (*Tadasana*): Stand evenly, either on your own or with hands resting on a chair back. Be especially aware of the sensation of the floor beneath you. Lift the toes, spread them wide, and press them into the floor. Spread the weight evenly through the balls of the feet and the heels, with strength in the outsides of the feet and a slight lift in the arches. Ground into the support of the floor while lengthening through the whole body and deepening the breath. Be aware of the action at your abdomen and draw it in slightly as you exhale, feeling the engagement of the core as you do so.

2. Perform brief joint movements to warm and loosen the ankles, knees, hips, ribs, wrists, elbows, and shoulders. Lean the head side to side and look right and left. You might shake out the arms and legs to increase circulation and sense of enlivenment.

3. Goddess Pose (*Deviasana*): Widen the stance with the knees straight but soft, rotate outward at the hips about 45 degrees or to your comfort. Gradually bend the knees, ensuring that they track over the ankles (you may need to widen the stance even more and/or reduce the angle), and feel the engagement of the thigh muscles. Continue pressing toward the outer edges of the feet, as rolling toward the instep puts uneven pressure through the knee joints. Hands can be on hips or shoulders or in cactus arms. Lengthen through the spine and feel empowered, with inner strength and energy as well as muscular strength.

4. Warrior Pose II (*Virabhadrasana II*): Rotate the hips back to parallel and extend the arms out to both sides. Step the feet almost as wide apart as the hands are. Turn the right toes out approximately 90 degrees (rotating from the hip) and the left toes are turned in slightly (about 45 degrees). Be mindful of how the knees are tracking over the ankles as you bend into the right knee, pressing into the outside of the right foot. Gaze over the right shoulder. Hands can be on hips, holding a chair back for support, or extending out to each side at shoulder height or lower. No matter what your arms are doing, feel a broadening across the chest and upper back.

Feel the support of the core as you stand tall and strong. Remember, as you feel your legs supporting you and your heart opening in your broad chest, that a part of strength is letting others support you and asking for/ receiving their kindness into your brave heart. Return to center and repeat this pose on the other side.

5. Return to center and find Mountain Pose. Take a few full, deep breaths and feel clarity of your open mind. Notice the earth beneath your feet again, feeling strong and stable. Acknowledge the effects of this practice on body, breath, emotions, and mind. Thank yourself for taking this time to strengthen the body and remind yourself of your inner strength in mind, emotions, and spirit.

POSTURE, CONCENTRATION: MINI-SEQUENCE FOR INNER PEACE

This sequence is designed to connect you to the subtler aspects of yourself, in service of a greater sense of peace. As such, the movements are smaller and attention is drawn deeper into the body. Although these cues are given for a person on the floor, you can connect to the intention of the postures while seated in a chair or standing up:

1. Begin in *Savasana*, propped as described in the Restorative Sequence in the previous chapter, with props for support and comfort as needed. Feel your breath deepen as you relax into the pose. Trust the earth to hold you so that your muscles can release completely. Let yourself be curious with the areas that are slower to relax, encouraging them to do so. Enjoy the chance to let go.

2. Pelvic Rocking: Place the soles of the feet on the floor at hip-width apart or slightly wider, about one foot away from the hips. Keep the knees in line with the hips and feet. If this is not comfortable for the knees, step the feet further away from the hips. On an exhale, press the natural curve of the lower back toward the floor; on an inhale, arch the back to exaggerate that curve. Move slowly between those two positions, noticing the places the back of your body is being massaged. Keep the breath long so that the

movement is very slow and intentional. Feel the effect of the movement up the length of the spine. After a few repetitions at a comfortable range of motion, see how small and subtle you can make the movement.

3. Stick Pose (*Yastikasana*): Extend both legs to return to your *Savasana* pose, feeling energy extend out the soles of both feet. If it is uncomfortable for the low back, place some support under the knees. As you inhale, reach your right arm forward and overhead as far as feels comfortable for the shoulder. Exhale, bring it back to your side. Alternate this movement left and right for a few breaths. Let the pace of your slow, deep breath guide the movement, rather than letting the pace of your arm set the depth of the breath. Notice what it's like to move your arm so slowly. Experience the details of what happens in your shoulders. How do your elbows, wrists, fingers, ribs, pelvis, and lower joints respond? Is there a difference depending on where your arm is in the arc? Finish with a full stick pose: reach both arms overhead within your available range and stretch the legs out as long as possible without overarching the back. If it feels better, this can also be done with arms out to the sides, feeling the stretch from head to toes and fingertip to fingertip.

4. Knees-to-Chest Pose (*Apanasana*): Draw both knees toward your chest and hold on behind the knees (holding on below the knees puts too much pressure on the knee joint). The legs can be together or hip-distance apart. If you can't comfortably reach the legs, place a strap or necktie behind the thighs and hold onto either end, drawing it toward you. If this doesn't feel good for the hips, rest the lower legs on the seat of a chair with the knees stacked over the hip joints. Let the lower legs relax into the posture. For an active experience, you can flex the feet and press through the heels, keeping the knees bent. You may use abdominal strength draw in the belly and bring your nose toward your knees (if that feels okay for the neck), keeping the chest broad and arms passive. This posture is associated with the flow through PMK that moves energies down and out of the body. When you exhale, imagine yourself releasing anything unnecessary from your body, emotions, and mind, as if they were flowing down your legs and out your feet. Everything that is not like peace blows away.

5. Bridge Pose (*Setu Bandhasana*): Place the soles of the feet on the floor, feet and knees at hip-width apart. As you inhale, press slowly and firmly into

the feet and lift the tailbone off of the floor. Pause and feel the strength through the lower legs, gluteals, and core. Exhale and release down to the floor. Repeat a few times, coming up higher if it feels comfortable. You might lift the sacrum and even the lower back off the floor. You can use a supported version of this pose, placing a pillow or block under the sacrum and staying here for a few breaths. Feel grounded and supported through the low body, free and open through the upper body. Notice any changes to the breath in this position. Roll down slowly as if one vertebrae at a time were reaching the floor.

6. Reclined Side Bend (*Bananasana*): Stretch out on your mat again. Imagine yourself like a fine sliver of moon in dark, peaceful sky. Exaggerate the stretch through the right side, bringing whole your body into a slight side curve. Enjoy long, energizing inhales and relax into the pose with each exhale. Return to center and stay in *Savansana* for a few breaths, sensing the difference between right and left side then repeat the stretch on the other side. Be sure to relax in *Savasana* after both sides, visualizing the peaceful moon and feeling calm vitalization.

7. Reclined Twist (*Supta Ardha Matsyendrasana*): Plant the feet wide apart on the floor with the knees bent toward the ceiling. Begin to slowly lower both knees to one side, then the other, exhaling as you lower and inhaling as you return to center. You may want a cushion or pillow on either side of the legs for support and/or between the knees. Let the breath set the pace for this action so it is unhurried and controlled. If it feels comfortable for the neck, you may want to turn your head gently in the opposite direction from the knees, creating a fuller twist through the spine. Stay at the minimum edge of sensation, so you perceive only a light stretch through the body. Set your focus on how good it feels to roll through the limbs, spine, and head with a soft smile.

8. Side Fetal Pose (*Parsva Garbhasana*): Curl up on your side as described in Step 3 of the Restorative Sequence of the previous chapter, with a cushion under the head and/or between the knees for comfort. Watch your breath deepen. Witness the ways in which your body relaxes as you bring your focus inward. Enjoy the process of letting go and create more space for a subtle, pervasive sense of peace.

9. Easy Pose (*Sukhasana*): When you are ready, use the support of your arms to return to any comfortable seated position. You may want to close the eyes, feeling the length in the spine, ease in the breath, and clarity in the mind. Keep these sensations with you as you acknowledge the effects of this sequence and carry on with your peaceful day.

This practice is designed to be rejuvenating and connect you to a deep sense of peace. Although there are only a few poses, if you take your time with this tranquil journey, the practice can last 90 minutes or longer. The small, exploratory actions give you permission to move very gently and bring a greater sense of ease and relaxation to your nervous system. Once you have completed the practice, be sure to notice the many opportunities for and gifts of peace throughout your day.

Summary

This chapter offered a variety of sequences for various intentions and abilities. Please return to these sequences as much as you'd like and pay attention to any changes in physical ability, breath, mood, coping, relationships, and outlook. Yoga affects us on all these levels and more. On days when even these brief routines are too lengthy or intense, remember that any healthy movement, deep breath, and mindful awareness are valuable. Stretch, move side to side and through twists, notice your thoughts. Even a single deep breath can make a difference in one's physical and mental state. Any simple health-promoting practice is worth doing, such as connecting to intention, mobilizing your joints, or having a good sigh. The following chapter gives you more tips on bringing yoga into your life or the lives of your clients for greater benefit.

Chapter 13

WHERE TO GO FROM HERE

This book has provided some information about the challenges of life with arthritis in its various forms, both in general terms and through the experiences of specific people. We have discussed the ways yoga may benefit the whole person with arthritis from a BPSS perspective. You have learned how poses, breathing exercises, relaxation, meditation, and perspective might affect quality of life on the physical, energetic, emotional, mental, and spiritual levels. There are a variety of experiential opportunities throughout the book. Our hope is that this book continues to benefit you, your clients, or those you love for years. This chapter aims to support you or them in some possible next steps to gain more information and personalized yoga therapy experiences. Below are recommendations and cautions for finding a suitable yoga class and/or yoga therapist while reiterating the benefits yoga can bring to the lives of those with arthritis.

How Medical Professionals Can Support Patients' Yoga Practice

It is becoming more common for physicians, specialists, and complementary/alternative healthcare providers to refer their clients and patients to yoga. As the empirical evidence mounts about its BPSS benefits, it is often revealed as a supportive lifestyle option. On the Yoga for Arthritis website,[131] you can find an information page for clinicians that may be a helpful way to start the conversation about yoga. Many rheumatologists have misconceptions about yoga like my colleagues in Johns Hopkins Rheumatology initially did. For the safety of patients, it is important to cultivate clear understanding and proper guidance as patients increasingly engage in more diverse self-care options.

If you are a healthcare practitioner, here are some things to remember about recommending yoga to your patients/clients:

1. Both medicine and yoga are guided by the fundamental precept of non-harm (*primum non nocere* in medicine and *ahmisa* in yoga). While professionals in each camp may think the other irresponsible in the wielding of our practices, we ultimately want the optimal for those we serve. We simply use a different set of tools in that effort.

2. Evaluate the general health and overall endurance of your patient/client, as well as any comorbid cardiovascular and pulmonary disease or severe osteoporosis so that the patient, and by extension the yoga teacher, is aware of the risks to the heart, lungs, or of fracturing bones or breaking them in a fall.

3. Clearly identify vulnerable joints to the patient (e.g. joints with instability, at particular risk for injury, with limited mobility, active swelling, or underlying damage, and any joints that have been replaced) so that your client knows what to pay special attention to during postures and can inform the teacher about these particular precautions. In all of these cases, the patient should be aware of the need for caution and to avoid positions that include movements contra-indicated after joint replacement or other surgery.

4. Clients are to be advised to listen to their bodies throughout class, avoiding movements that exacerbate pain. Additionally, it should be a standard of behavior that they review any possible problem areas and limitations with the instructor prior to starting the class.

5. You may consider providing a letter for the yoga instructor, outlining general and specific medical and musculoskeletal concerns. Care providers can also agree to speak directly with the yoga instructor and provide a contact number.

6. Engage in ongoing dialogue with your client regarding yoga experience and concerns. Review warning signs of injury and appropriate management of discomfort (e.g. rest, apply cold/heat). It is also an option to refer your patient to a physical and/or occupational therapist for assessment of limitations and required modifications. This further review is a stepping stone to safe and fruitful yoga practice.

7. If you have any questions about yoga, seek out a yoga therapist in your area to interview, contact one of the many accredited training facilities, or reach out to me and my colleagues at Yoga for Arthritis. We are happy to support your work and the wellbeing of your patients.

Yoga for Arthritis *Sutras*

For those readers teaching yoga to people with arthritis, these "threads" (*sutras*), when practiced together, weave a safe, enjoyable class. Note your habits as a teacher—the ones you implement easily and the ones you need to work on.

Model the simplest version of the pose

Students see you as an expert. Whatever version of the pose you model will be seen as "correct," "valid," or "real." If you model the most accessible version, it gives students the freedom to feel comfortable making that choice. Additionally, some students may not be able to hear you and will be following your movements. You want to make sure such students are safe. If students have a more advanced practice, they will know the classical version of the pose and can use it. I often demonstrate several variations for a moment each (e.g. "You can place your hands here, here, or here") and then return to the simplest option. Otherwise, I verbally explain other choices (e.g. "Your foot can stay here, come to the calf, or up to the thigh") while staying in a simple variation.

Use inclusive non-hierarchical language

Students with arthritis often feel "less than" due to their limitations. If one student is sitting in a chair and the others are standing, I will be sure that my verbal instruction includes the person in the chair. I will explain the pose in the chair first, so they knows what to do before guiding the standing students. I will often sit in the chair and model while using verbal instruction for the standers. Additionally, all pose options should be presented as a buffet, not a hierarchy. There are no levels in Yoga for Arthritis, only options. Like a buffet, no one option is better than any of the others. They are all just options. The cantaloupe is not better than the pineapple; it's just a different choice. Our language goes a long way to putting those choices on an even playing field so that students are making appropriate selections based on how they feel, not on a notion of which version they think is objectively better.

Make sure everyone is breathing

I mean this partly in a literal sense. Oftentimes, students will stop breathing when in concentration or striving for a posture. If they are not able to breathe normally, they are not in an appropriate posture. Some might even say that if they are not breathing, it isn't yoga. But beyond just breathing, every class should include attention to the breath. This includes integrating breath with movements, bringing awareness back to the breath and introducing specific *pranayama* practices. Some have called *pranayama* the "secret sauce" of yoga—what makes it different from exercise or other physical modalities. On a physiological level, it alters nervous system function and improves cellular repair (much needed in the context of chronic disease). Use it to its fullest.

Don't face away from your students or close your eyes

This might seem obvious, but I've seen it many times. Some teachers turn away from students because mirroring is complicated. You don't have to mirror. Everyone in the room doesn't have to be doing the same side at once as long as everyone gets to both sides. Not all yoga professionals feel this way, but I think safety and attending to our students trump doing the left side first. You can also use landmarks in the room (e.g. the side closest to the windows). While closing your eyes might help you check into your own energetic state or soften your voice, it is more important to know what is happening for your students. In fact, just seeing is not even enough.

In Chinese, the word "listen" includes the characters for eyes, ears, attention, and heart. Try to bring all of those aspects to the way you listen and attend to your students. Your primary responsibility as a teacher is to be clued into how they are doing at all times.

Ensure appropriate student–teacher ratio

In order to truly "see" everyone in the room, you might need to have fewer people in the room. Start out with four or six at most. As you build skills of awareness and attentiveness, this may increase. Consider bringing in an assistant to serve as another set of eyes, ears, and guiding hands. Some large Yoga for Arthritis classes have two assistants. If you find yourself teaching to a large group and it is not possible to attend to everyone, consider keeping everyone seated. I have taught to stadiums that way and no one got hurt. It is possible to have a fully engaging and physically comprehensive class in the safety of a chair.

Stay within your scope of practice and refer as appropriate

Do you know your scope of practice? There is an official scope of practice established by the International Association of Yoga Therapists that can serve as a guide. It is safe to say that your scope of practice is limited to the tools of yoga, which happen to be fairly robust. Never give advice that is outside of that scope. It is unethical and in some cases illegal. When students see you as an expert, they may ask questions that you are not authorized to answer. Many yoga teachers also know a lot about other therapeutic modalities, but unless you are a licensed professional and serving in that capacity, refer students to someone who is. You may even want to refer a student to another yoga professional who has training and expertise in an area that would best serve them. Sending a student to another professional when indicated is a practice of *ahimsa* and foundational to yoga itself.

Maintain confidentiality

While this is aligned with the *yamas* and *niyamas*, it is also an ethical tenant in most health-related fields. Even if you are not legally bound by confidentiality laws (i.e. HIPAA), it is professional and ethically appropriate to act as if you were. Treat all personal and health information in the highest confidence, protecting both spoken words and written documents. This also applies within your classes. Do not assume that students are comfortable sharing their diagnosis or other health information with fellow students, and certainly you should not make such information public without explicit permission. Confidentiality should extend beyond diagnoses and health information to any personal information shared directly or indirectly, unless told otherwise. There are some exceptions to privacy laws, such as an intention to harm self or others. *Ahimsa* comes into play here, but you should know the relevant laws and procedures in your region and for similar professions.

Never skip meditation

Meditation literally grows the brain, particularly in regions affected by chronic pain. It can change pain pathways and alter emotional reactivity to the experience of pain. Meditation also makes it easier to maintain equanimity in the face of pain, however it changes. Skipping meditation is a disservice to your students at the very least. There are many types of meditation and some may be more accessible to students than others. Consider focusing on the breath or something with personal meaning. Try a mindfulness meditation or loving kindness. Use a walking meditation or a guided meditation. This goes for each of the other aspects of yoga, too (relaxation, centering, philosophy, etc.). Don't leave anything out. Your students deserve the range of benefits that each of the yoga practices fosters.

Explain the science

You don't have to be a scientist to tell students that building quadriceps strength stabilizes the knee joint. You don't need a PhD to explain that slow exhales calm the nervous system. You don't have to be a neuroscientist to tell them that meditation grows grey matter in the brain. Science helps students to understand why these practices can help them to manage arthritis better. Science also helps them explain it to others. It might even help them to visualize the changes in their own bodies, which can bring its own benefits. Don't spend the whole class focused on science lessons but mention a few concepts in each class. Just be sure when doing so that your science is correct!

Consistently integrate philosophy

In my experience, it is not the physical effects of yoga that are usually most profound for students; it is the way they change their mindset, their life choices and their relationships to body and disease. Bring in the *yamas* and *niyamas*. Talk about a pose as a metaphor for life. Mention how students can take a practice off the mat and into other contexts. You are providing tools for living differently, not just a temporary escape from the challenges of life.

Honor and foster the absolute autonomy of your students

Each of your students is the world's leading expert of their own body. I provide verbal cues or even light touch with permission to guide alignment, but I never move a student into a posture. I allow them to proceed with awareness, knowing their limits better than I ever will. Similarly, I honor their choices throughout the class. Hopefully, this can empower students to feel more in charge of their own bodies and their own lives in other contexts. Outside expertise is important and useful, but, ultimately, students get to decide what is best for them.

Never stop learning

Insights, lessons, new ideas, and deeper understanding come from students, teachers, ancient wisdom, modern science, personal practice, and beyond. Keep searching.

Finding Your Own Yoga for Arthritis Class

It is up to the person with arthritis to decide how the yoga will begin. Whether you have RA or OA, or some other form of systemic or inflammatory condition, it is ideal to start with live instruction by a qualified and experienced professional, in a setting where individual guidance and feedback is available. Only a live teacher can observe and provide feedback about how to safely execute the poses. After some training (or in between classes), you may want to start practicing yoga at home. As with any physical activity, speak with your rheumatologist, orthopedist, or other medical provider(s) about whether it is appropriate for you, given your unique situation.

Many of my clients and students admit that they wanted to take yoga for many years before actually attending a class. A number of concerns stood in their way:

thoughts about safety; looking stupid, incapable, or different; fear of injury or making the condition worse; or seeing contortionist postures in the media and thinking that was how to practice yoga. These are valid concerns, as some forms of yoga do pressure students to perform postures in a regimented way, which is not appropriate for arthritis. Yoga classes for arthritis require modification and a non-judgmental approach. Some yoga classes incorporate extreme positions and not all teachers are aware of why or how to modify the *asanas*. I understand why you might have concerns about practicing yoga.

People do get hurt practicing yoga. The typical ways people get hurt are through extreme class environments (such as excess heat, regimented technique, or a competitive philosophy), not being given options/modifications for postures, moving quickly between postures so there is little time for awareness and adaptation, or pushing too hard. That is not the kind of yoga I recommend. The good news is that with a few simple questions, you can screen out the unsuitable classes and find a class and teacher that meets the needs of a person with arthritis.

The steps to finding a suitable yoga class are:

1. Speak with your healthcare team and receive clearance from your doctor(s) to participate in yoga.

2. Research the classes available in your area.

3. Have a phone conversation with the people at the studio and ask the questions listed below.

4. Arrive early to a class and talk to the teacher before it starts.

5. Be the authority of your body during class. Listen to yourself and do not overextend.

6. Observe the effect of class on your whole self for the next few days.

Step 1: Check with Your Doctor

Before beginning any fitness regime or marked lifestyle change, it is important that your healthcare team is involved in the process. In general, people looking after your wellbeing will be pleased about the incorporation of a fitness and stress reduction program. Often, they will make you aware of any specific concerns or movements to avoid.

Sometimes, doctors will recommend avoiding yoga and this could be for one of two reasons: 1) The doctor does not know much about yoga and fears you will be asked to perform physical feats that will strain the joints; or 2) The patient's arthritis or physical functioning are not in a place where beginning an activity program is advisable.

To address the first issue, offer to provide the doctor with literature about the research behind the program and examples of the gentle poses involved in the practice. You can even suggest that the doctor call the yoga center to discuss it in more detail. However, if the second issue is involved, it is not advisable for you to participate until your health or functioning recover. In the meantime, you may begin interacting with yoga by performing some of the personal reflections, relaxations, and gentle breathing exercises in this book. Do whatever physical activity the doctor recommends, such as a short daily walk, and hopefully yoga will be an option when the disease stabilizes.

Step 2: Research the Classes in Your Area

There are numerous types of yoga classes that may be suitable for a person with arthritis. If you live in a small town with limited options, seek out a "gentle," "restorative," "beginner," or "therapeutic" class. If you have significant limitations or trouble getting to the floor, consider starting with a "chair yoga" class. "Yoga for Seniors" is a good option even if you are a young person because of the humor, compassion, and accepting approach evident in those classes. These teachers tend to have greater experience in modifying postures and may be better able to support you in finding a safe and more comfortable position. Additionally, they will support your beginning needs and a slower pace. Even a "*hatha*," "Classical," or "Integral" Yoga class with a teacher who supports modifications could be a good fit. In the best of circumstances, you may find a Yoga for Arthritis class.

Just a few years ago, it may have been hard to find a yoga teacher specializing in arthritis. Today, there are several approaches to find a good fit for yourself or your clients/patients. I have trained over a hundred teachers in Yoga for Arthritis and offer continuing education for yoga teachers specifically about arthritis. You can find some of those teachers featured on our website at www.arthritis.yoga or contact us for a recommendation in your area. Some yoga teachers also have a healthcare background that provides useful context about life with these conditions. In fact, you might even find a yoga teacher who has been living with arthritis or a related condition for many years themselves.

If you are struggling with where to begin, please contact the Yoga for Arthritis organization for additional guidance. We are happy to support you as you explore available group classes. It is important to start slowly and mindfully, with a teacher who can offer skillful guidance for safety and optimal outcomes.

Vicki Finds Her Teacher

It can take some time to find the class and teacher who connects with you and offers yoga in a way that fits your needs and beliefs. Vicki suffers from fibromyalgia, myofascial pain syndrome, and piriformis pain syndrome, in addition to OA. She has arthritis in both knees, both hands, and both feet which also affects her cervical, lumbar, and sacral vertebrae. She has five bulging discs in her neck and three in the low back due to degeneration of the discs:

> It's a typical story: there are calcium deposits and pressure on my trunk nerves which cause stiffness, cramping, and radicular nerve pain that particularly affects my neck, back, hips, and legs. I went pain clinic where I was a frequent flyer for epidural shots—transforaminal epidural injections—to the spinal nerves with massive doses of steroids to control my misery. It had gotten to the point of needing them nearly once a year to control the pain. In between, the chiropractor's office was used to seeing me on a regular basis to keep symptoms in check ranging from the tip of neck to the base of my spine. In between, I was fairly miserable. I was taking a fair amount of opiate medications, as well. Symptoms first appeared when I was only 17 years old and only got worse and worse to the age of 60.

Vicki kept herself fit and mobile with water aerobics until the class was cancelled:

> I wondered, *How I am going to get some exercise?* At a visit to my chiropractor's office, I learned that the yoga instructor Sandy Palmer was going to start holding classes there. I decided to give it a shot. I contacted Sandy and began taking yoga classes twice per week. Sandy was wonderful. She started me out on my yoga practices very slowly and gently. She reminded me on a regular basis not to do anything that hurt so that I would in no way injure myself or cause any exacerbations of my symptoms. It went slowly as

I became stronger and more flexible. Yoga became a regular and pleasurable part of my life.

I went from someone who could not bend over and touch my fingertips to the ground to someone who can nearly lay my hands flat on the floor. Amazing! Now at age 65, I am doing yoga postures that I could never have imagined or aspired to. I am healthier and happier than I have been in all of my adult life. My advice to anyone with neck, back, or radiating nerve pain—take up yoga and practice it regularly.

I was fortunate to have found Sandy. She has guided me to be what I consider to be a fairly well-accomplished yoga practitioner. I won't claim my arthritis has been cured, but my pain and stiffness are 100 per cent improved. I have not even considered having an epidural injection in my spinal nerves for five years. I rarely find the need to see my chiropractor. And, I rarely need to take a pain pill. Yoga has been a success story for me. I hope others will read this and pursue this lifestyle change that has worked so well for me.

Step 3: Looking Into a Yoga Center

Once you have researched your options for yoga classes, it is best to call each facility and ask questions about their teachers, standards and approach. The following is a sample list of questions. Your doctor, rheumatologist, and other healthcare providers may also alert you to specific concerns—unique to you—that you might want to ask about. Be sure to identify up front that you are interested in yoga due to your arthritis so that the person answering your questions can best describe how their offerings might support you.

Are you a registered yoga teacher or certified yoga therapist? Please tell me about your training.

Yoga Alliance is the recognition body for yoga instructors worldwide. Being registered with Yoga Alliance requires a minimum level of training in techniques, anatomy/physiology, teaching methodology, philosophy/ethics, and practical experience. While there are still many differences between training programs, due to the diversity of yoga traditions and approaches, there is a core industry standard.

Most yoga teachers working today are trained at least at the 200-hour level and many receive the additional 300 hours to be a 500-hour yoga teacher.

In the emerging field of yoga therapy, the International Association of Yoga Therapists (IAYT) requires a minimum of 1,000 hours of training and experience working with clinical populations such as those with arthritis or other pain conditions. The IAYT accredits training programs and certifies yoga therapists as C-IAYTs.

How long have you been teaching?

While this is not always the case, teachers with more experience are often more adept at modifying poses for each individual. They have had years to work with a variety of students and have likely made many discoveries about individual differences and potential adaptations during that time. Additionally, they might have continued training for students with special needs, conditions, or health concerns.

Do you have a medical/healthcare background or experience teaching students with arthritis?

This is an ideal scenario. Many yoga instructors decided to teach because they discovered the healing properties of yoga through their own journeys. It is not unusual for someone in the healthcare field to teach yoga because of the range of benefits it provides. Even if they do not come from a medical background, try to find a teacher who is familiar with your condition and can guide you in making the proper adjustments for your body. Short of this, classes offered through hospitals or medical settings are often supervised or overseen by medical staff and may be a good option for you.

How do you teach your classes?

Based on your research, you are calling places that offer some form of yoga that seems like it might benefit your arthritis symptoms. Confirm at the beginning of the call that they do offer that style (gentle, restorative, beginner, *hatha*, chair, senior, etc.). Each may do the practices with slightly different form or in a different order, emphasizing different aspects. Many modern classes draw from a variety of styles to best suit the general population or people who tend to go to classes in that space. If you have taken yoga classes before, you may encounter some things that are familiar and some that are quite different. Ultimately, this is your journey and for safety and comfort, you will make the poses your own.

I have numerous movement limitations. Will I be the only one in class changing how I perform the postures?

It is actually okay if you are the only one. Some people feel nervous or singled out by being the only person who modifies poses and sequences; however, soon enough they realize that no one else in the class is bothered by it (it may even inspire some people!) and the class itself, not just the teacher, becomes a source of support. This question elicits a general tone about how much you will be encouraged to adapt your practice. As the instructor answers, listen for the ways s/he will accept your limitations and help you adapt the class to suit your specific needs. Gain a sense of how much diversity happens within the class and the level of encouragement the teacher transmits. The ideal is "a lot"!

What kinds of props do you have available and how much do you use them?

There is a range in the amount and kinds of props available and how much teachers utilize them. Yoga props are incredibly useful for students with arthritis. For example, I use a yoga wedge (a less common prop) for any postures that require weight bearing in the hands. I also put a folded blanket under my knees for cushioning during floor poses. If props aren't available, there are other adjustments to make with the position of various body parts for greater ease or comfort. As you practice and work with your teacher, you will find the adjustments and props that work best for your body. Once you figure out what works for you, you can take that knowledge into any yoga class! The next couple of questions address adjustments and modifications.

I can't sit on the floor. Are there other ways I can do the postures?

Some students may have a difficult time getting up and down from the floor. One big reason for this is that putting weight on their knees is painful, even for the moment of transition from standing to sitting. You also may not be very strong, flexible, or physically fit (yet!), which can impede the ability to sit on the floor. Hopefully, your yoga teacher will work with you to find a tolerable method, such as one of those mentioned in this book. Putting a folded blanket or bolster below your knee can help, or even offering hands for assistance. Leaning on a chair or the wall can help you feel more stable. However, when we focus on the intention underlying a pose, we can also adapt any *asana* for a different orientation such as sitting on a chair or lying on the floor. Hopefully, your new yoga teacher will be helpful and encouraging so that after a period of time using the wall or chair to reorient a pose, you become comfortable with moving up and down from the floor. This skill can also benefit you in other areas of life.

My ankle (or knee, back, etc.) doesn't bend like that. Do I have any options?

Especially if you have been living with arthritis for many years, you may have fused joints or had joint replacement surgery. These naturally impose limitations. Sometimes, moving joints in a particular way can be very painful. It is more important to be minimize pain and remain comfortable than it is to do the pose in a traditional way. Your yoga teacher should work with you to find a position that suits you better but still honors the essence of the pose and challenges you in some way.

It hurts to put weight on my hands. Are there other things I can do?

This is a common complaint for people with arthritis in their hands or wrists. In fact, some people are unable to put their hands on the ground due to deformities or bone fusion. It can be especially challenging for postures like Table, Downward-Facing Dog, or Plank. You may want to use a wedge to change the wrist angle, use blocks that the fingers can hang over, make fists, or do the pose on a chair or against the wall so you can reduce weight in the hands. Similarly, you might try Cobra with hands hovering above the floor or without any pressure in the hands, even if they are still on the floor.

How many people attend your classes?

Most class sizes range from five to 25 people. You decide how many people you are comfortable practicing with. A smaller group means more individual attention.

If there are a large number of people in the class you are considering, you may ask the follow-up question,

How do you ensure the safety of such a big class?

Be sure to check in with your healthcare team about any other questions you should be asking and if curiosities arise during the conversation, ask those questions, too. Ensure you have asked all of your questions before attending the class, even if it means calling back again. That said, do not procrastinate going to yoga. If you get there and you feel that it is not a good fit, you can decide to leave and look elsewhere.

Is Hot Yoga Good for Arthritis?

There are many people with arthritis who feel intense symptoms in cold weather and find relief in warmth. There are some who experience the opposite. There is a difference between a warm room and a hot room. Hot rooms may not be appropriate for those who are new to yoga, lacking fitness, or at risk of overheating. Hot rooms may also bring an increase in pathogens that can be of concern for those on immune-suppressing medications. Additionally, hot rooms increase flexibility. This may seem like a good thing, but it can result in overstretching. For someone who has an advanced yoga practice and is able to work within appropriate limits, a warm room might feel good. It should be noted, though, that some yoga practices in hot rooms are vigorous, intense, and/or fast-paced, which is likely to be less safe for those with joint disease who require the time and ease to pay attention and adapt the practice as it progresses. While both yoga and warmth are often soothing for aches and pains, extreme environments are inherently risky.

Step 4: Attending a New Class

It can be scary to start anything new, especially as an adult. You may have been living with the pain of arthritis for a long time and feel apprehensive about physical activity that could further injure you. Remember that you are the expert of your own body and you will not perform anything that causes you pain. That being said, starting a new physical activity can be a challenge, so be prepared for working some muscles you may have forgotten about. Give yourself the freedom to experiment with attending a few different classes to get a sense of what your local options are for studios, styles, and teachers.

When you start a new class, try to arrive early so that you have enough time for a conversation with the teacher. Explain that you have arthritis, which type it is and how it affects you symptomatically. Tell the teacher which joints are involved, how your movement might be limited and any movements that cause joint pain. Even if they doesn't know much about arthritis, you can probably work together to find appropriate modifications. Ask if there is a posture you should return to in case you can't figure out how to modify the one being taught or you need a break (and make sure it's something that doesn't hurt!). If the teacher isn't willing/able to help you find different ways to execute a pose, which s/he should be after the telephone conversation, find another teacher.

Step 5: Participate within Your Limits

During yoga practice, avoid anything that causes additional pain to the joints. If you feel any sensation that is sharp or shooting, back off and ask for an alternative variation to the pose. Remember the resting alternative the teacher provided from your conversation in class. Perform it when in doubt.

One of the reasons yoga works well for rheumatoid conditions is that it can be adapted to work for each person. *Do not go further into a pose that increases your pain.* You will feel the sensation of gently stretching and toning muscles, but that should be in the thickest part of the muscle, not at the joint. Be sure to keep the recommendations of your healthcare team in mind, perhaps even bringing notes from your medical provider to the first few yoga classes. You are the authority of your body during class. Respect the teacher but choose for yourself. Listen to obvious and subtle messages from your body and do not overextend.

Step 6: Observe the Effects of Class

The effects of a yoga class may be evident for days after the practice. Remember that yoga is not just a physical activity. It is a holistic mindfulness practice that includes a variety of components (deep breathing, relaxation, meditation, visualization, concentration, etc.). As with any physical activity, you may also experience some soreness after yoga practice. This comes from using muscles in a new way. Following the guidelines of your healthcare team and listening to your body during class can help limit this, but it will also diminish in time as your fitness improves. Be sure to drink plenty of water during and after practice. You may also want to gently stretch any sore muscles or take a warm bath. If discomfort is severe or if it persists for more than two days, contact your rheumatologist. You may want to plan for a less active day after your first few yoga practices, until you get acclimated to this new activity. Other effects are also evident right away. Anecdotally, people sometimes report improved sleep after just one class, a greater capacity for breath or increased sense of optimism. You might consider starting a journal to track the benefits that you notice over time, physically, energetically, emotionally, mentally, and spiritually. You can also use this to document any questions that arise about yoga for your yoga teacher or for your doctor.

Table 13.1: Yoga Therapy Benefits the Whole Person with Arthritis

Kosha	Potential Benefits of Yoga Therapy and Yoga for Arthritis Classes
Body (*annamaya kosha*)	Increased strength/Slowed muscle loss
	Increased mobility
	Increased physical endurance and fitness
	Weight loss, which reduces pressure on joints and the role of excess fat in inflammation
	Reduced pain
	Reduced joint swelling/inflammation
	Increased joint lubrication
	Improved balance (help prevent falls)
	Strengthened tissues around the joints to stabilize them
Energy (*pranamaya kosha*)	Increased energy
	Balance of autonomic nervous system and other systems
	Greater quality of rest
Mind (*manomaya kosha*)	Greater focus
	Improved sleep
	Decreased depressive symptoms
	Decreased anxiousness
	Improved mood
	Better stress management

cont.

Kosha	Potential Benefits of Yoga Therapy and Yoga for Arthritis Classes
Intellect (*vijnanamaya kosha*)	Greater ability to relax and respond, rather than react, to life
	Improved outlook
	Increased body awareness
	More awareness of and adaptation to ever-changing mental/emotional and physical needs
	Greater acceptance of limitations, enhanced self-efficacy for disease management, and greater self-care
Spiritual (*anandamaya kosha*)	Improved perceptions of overall wellbeing
	Potential to receive positive regard from a community
	Inspiration through relationships with others who are active and thriving with arthritis
	Understanding from those who understand the particular pains of rheumatoid conditions
	Improved self-care (nutrition, rest, fitness, time for self, medical adherence, community connections, service, etc.)
	More engagement in life, activities, relationships, and service
	Connection to the deepest aspects of oneself
	Value and awareness of the most important things in life

Yoga Therapy

For a more intimate and individualized yoga experience, you may want to work with a yoga therapist. Yoga therapists generally work one-on-one with individuals or small groups that focus on a particular condition or concern. Yoga therapists often have more training than most yoga teachers (1,000 hours total) and they tend to specialize in working with individual needs/limitations. This can be an especially good place to start if you have a lot of movement limitations, multiple health concerns, or any trepidation about a more standard group class experience. The International Association of Yoga Therapists has established standards for training yoga therapists and accredits programs worldwide. Yoga therapy is a wonderful way to get yourself into a yoga practice because you will experience a tailored and evolving plan of care for the session and daily life that is customized for your unique condition and priorities.

Just as you had a series of questions for a potential yoga teacher, so you may similarly want to interview your yoga therapist. Once again, be sure to ask any yoga therapists what their training includes, what their approach is and how much experience they have with arthritis in particular. A yoga therapist will weave postures, breathing, relaxation, and meditation with yoga philosophy to support you in creating a lifestyle of health and wellbeing. Yoga therapists are practiced at approaching their work based on the PMK model, so they will put effort toward balancing all levels of your being and offering practices that leverage the interactions of body, energy, emotions, mind, wisdom, and spirit. A yoga therapist who has been through a training accredited by the International Association of Yoga Therapists is likely to have sufficient skills and knowledge to meet the needs and limitations of arthritis.

While yoga therapy may be more expensive than a yoga class, it provides you the opportunity to learn safe ways to practice yoga at home, which is free, convenient, and can be carried with you for years to come. A yoga therapist can individualize a short practice that is appropriate for you in order to facilitate health on all levels. As part of your professional relationship, the yoga therapist will follow-up with you to find out how it is working and make adjustments as needed. If you get tired of the practice or need to make changes for any reason, you can return to the yoga therapist for a tune-up of your home practice. The intentions for yoga therapy may revolve around reducing or managing the range of symptoms that cause pain, including psychological. In addition to improving overall function and helping to prevent the underlying causes of the symptoms and disease, it can provide you with actionable steps toward improved health and wellbeing. Small group classes specifically targeted toward arthritis and chronic pain may seem more accessible as you continue working with a yoga therapist and many yoga therapists offer (or can recommend) specialized classes. With some practice, you may start to feel stronger and more comfortable and confident moving into a gentle or beginner class.

A yoga therapist has specialized training to work with physical limitations, pain conditions, as well as fatigue, sleep disruption, and the depressive symptoms that are common for people with arthritis. The yoga therapist will conduct a comprehensive intake to understand individual concerns and limitations, and will design a plan of care that is appropriate for a specific individual to implement. The first two limbs of yoga, the ethical principles of *yamas* and *niyamas*, guide the work of a yoga therapist and are reflected in a focus on self-care in everyday life. For example, the work day might become a practice of self-study and surrender while rest is a practice of non-harm and purity. Yoga practice is integrated at a higher level of being, where the practice is ongoing, no matter the physical condition or situation.

Yoga therapists are an excellent part of a comprehensive healthcare team. They are trained to work with medical professionals and other CIH providers. They consider each client as a whole person and will collaborate and advocate as needed when your concerns reach outside their professional scope. Typically, yoga therapists have a referral network so that if you require additional expertise or would benefit from a different kind of care, they can connect you to a trusted professional with those skills. You are the expert of your own body and the ultimate decision-maker regarding your healthy routines and care. Having a team of experts supporting you sets you up for optimum coping as you journey with arthritis.

REFLECTION: YOUR HEALTHCARE TEAM

This reflection exercise is to acknowledge the ways you have already built a team around you and identify opportunities to broaden or leverage your support network. Take some time to reflect upon and answer the following questions in your journal:

1. Who is part of your healthcare team already? (List medical and psychological professionals, as well as fitness and nutrition professionals, massage therapists, physical therapists, etc. You may also include supportive friends, family, neighbors, and even bloggers or authors who inspire you.)

2. List all of the many ways your care-team plan is helpful. Remember to consider yourself as a whole person, in body, energy, mind, wisdom, and spirit and identify the good these professional (or personal) relationships provide you.

3. What qualities does your team possess that make you feel supported?

4. Now consider any healthcare providers that have not been as helpful. What qualities or behaviors did they have that seemed to interfere with, limit, or delay your healing process on any level? Note, this is not about blaming or rehashing old problems, but is simply a means of noticing and learning from past experiences in order to optimize your care in the future.

5. Considering the quality of support and care you are currently receiving, what is important for you to remember as you seek further support, either from a yoga teacher, yoga therapist, or other health professional?

6. And perhaps most importantly, how will you remember to be your own best advocate?

Carry this exercise into your life by telling your care workers some of the things you appreciate about them (Step 3). Remember the answers to Step 6, especially when you find yourself in a new environment, working with a new care provider, or feeling in some way confused or unsure. Reaffirm your confidence and the right to advocate for yourself on a regular basis.

Summary

People choose to start yoga for many different reasons; however, the outcomes of the journey may be similar. According to research and one-on-one discussions with students over many years, we see that yoga can provide comfort for a sore, tired body. It may improve energy while still accommodating fatigue, teaching acceptance for things as they are and being highly adaptable so that there is always some form of practice available. Yoga offers space for whatever emotions and thoughts are present and gives us the chance to witness and consider a range of responses. The philosophical components provide a framework for life and offer context to stress, anxiety, depression, and other psychological aspects that are often magnified by chronic disease. Yoga classes can build social relationships and provide a consistently supportive environment for unwinding, relaxation, and even humor. Yoga can aid in managing the symptoms of arthritis, functional abilities, emotions, perspectives, relationships, self-esteem, and overall quality of life for the whole person.

Yoga can be an enjoyable way to stay active and help to manage rheumatic conditions as one of the safe and healthy non-pharmacological approaches to accompany state-of-the-art medical care available for arthritis. It is important, however, to begin the journey safely. This includes finding a qualified instructor, speaking to your medical providers and listening to your body. As you practice yoga over time, you may notice that it changes the way you stand, the way you breathe, even the way you see things. General quality of life has been shown to improve with yoga practice. People with arthritis also report a shift in perspective due to yoga practice, changing the relationship to the disease, themselves, or the body in general. These changes can be so profound that people speak of yoga as a way of life and a critical component of disease management, sometimes for decades after beginning the practice. Teaching participants how to adapt yoga poses for their unique abilities and limitations is a transferrable skill that brings acceptance and adaptability, other life activities, and experiences, too. I hope that this book will continue to support you and your clients in approaching yoga with safety and appreciation of yourself.

Appendix

Adapting and Modifying Postures

A: Centering

Start in a comfortable seated position. There are several options for this. Each knee can rest on the opposite lower leg, one leg can be in front of the other, or knees can rest on blocks/blankets for support. Do not offer half or full lotus for arthritis patients. If there is rounding in the lower back, suggest sitting on blocks or blankets to reduce the intensity of the stretch and make it easier to have a vertical spine. Sitting in a chair is another option, but if you are able, try sitting on the floor because getting up and down from the floor will build strength, confidence, and translate into practical life activities (like reaching into low kitchen cabinets or playing with kids on the floor!). Another option is to sit on a block with legs folded under, but it is important to make sure ankles are right under hips so the knee is not torqued. If there is knee pain in any of these positions, try additional modifications. It is fine to change position as necessary and sitting for longer periods will become more tolerable with time. Centering practices are outlined in Chapters 1, 8, and 11.

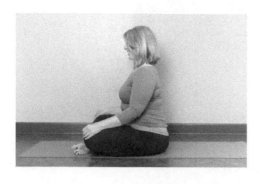
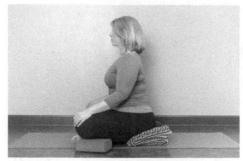
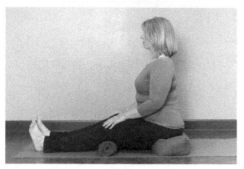
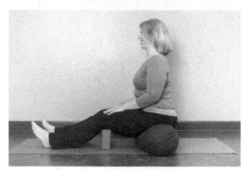

B: Warm-Up

The beginning of the warm up should be slow and easy, moving the spine in all three planes (forward bend/arch, side stretch, twist). You can vary them a bit each time you practice, according to how you feel. You may want to start with just the head, add the torso, then add the arms. This should all be done in a seated position just to loosen up the body. You can hold each for a little while, or you can repeat them, moving slowly from one to the next in a fluid motion. The idea is to start moving the major joints so that you can feel a bit less stiff and prepared for larger movements. Be sure to sit up tall and create length and space in the spine before any spinal movements.

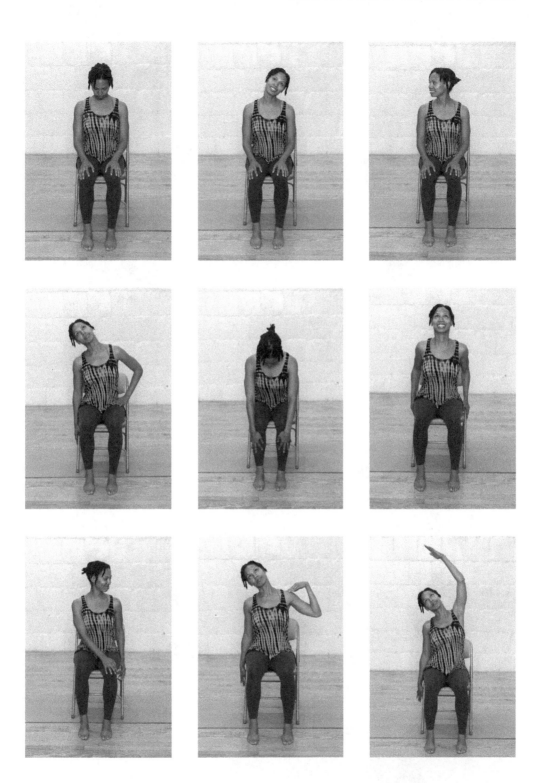

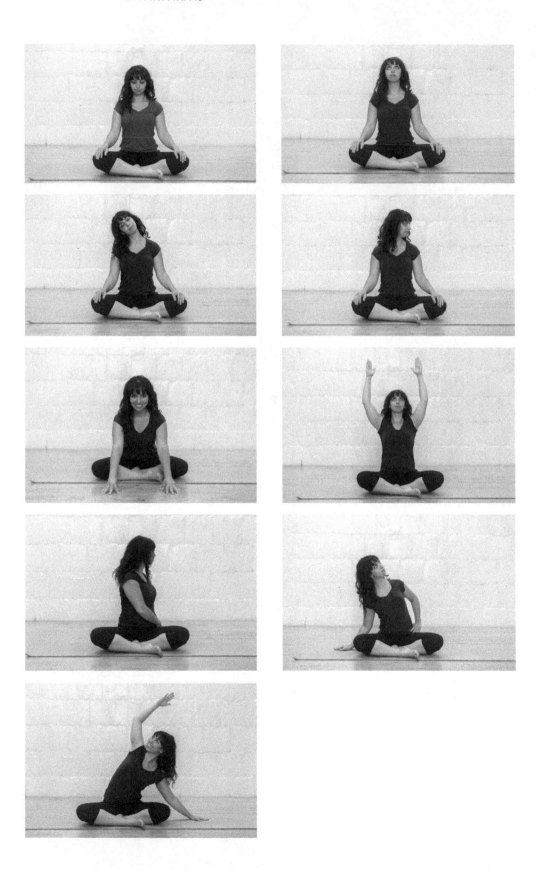

C: Hand and Wrist Variations

When weight-bearing you might support the wrists with a fold of the mat so that the end of the hand and fingers are off the mat and on the floor in front of you. This can also be accomplished with a folded blanket. If that isn't enough support, try a yoga wedge under the hands with the high side oriented so it decreases the wrist angle. You can also support your weight on the fingertips, fists, or forearms instead of the palms, keeping the shoulders integrated and avoiding locked elbows. Forearms should generally be on blocks or other props, depending on limb length, in order to maintain alignment. With forearms on blocks, the hands and wrists have no pressure and can be placed in any orientation. Moving poses from the floor to a chair or wall can also decrease the weight and pressure in the joints. If bringing palms together in prayer position is too much wrist extension, try touching the fingertips of each hand together and feeling the energy between the palms, make a fist with one hand and hold onto it with the other hand, or place the palms on the heart center. Instead of interlacing fingers with palms pressing away, interlace the fingers and press the backs of the hands away from the body instead, so that the wrists are in flexion and not extension. (For those with carpal tunnel syndrome, many of these variations may need to be reversed, so it's important to listen to your body and respond accordingly.)

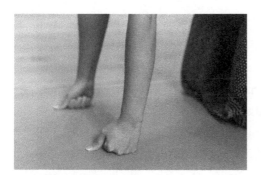 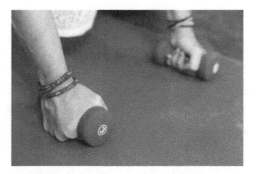

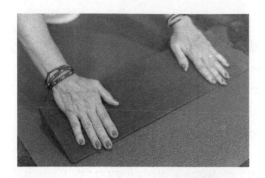

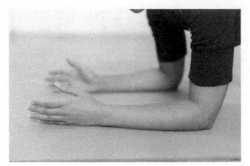

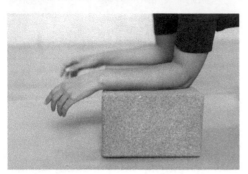

D: Hands and Knees Postures

a: Table

Come to the hands and knees, perhaps with a folded blanket under the knees for cushioning. Knees should be hip-distance apart, with thighs perpendicular to the floor. Elbows are under the shoulders. Palms can be flat on the floor or on a wedge. Alternatively, you can tent the fingers, make fists, or rest the forearms on blocks. If you are working to build upper body strength, this might become tiring quickly. Don't hesitate to rest as needed and re-enter the pose. With time, you may want to try challenging your balance by extending an arm or leg. This can be done statically or dynamically with the breath. For a greater challenge, you can try extending one arm and the opposite leg simultaneously. Feel a long line of energy reaching out in both directions. It's okay to wobble as your strength and balance improves.

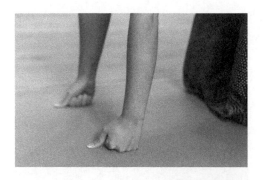
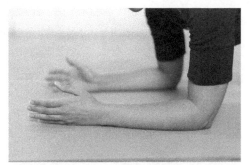
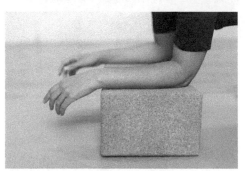
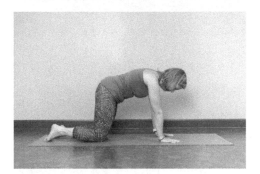
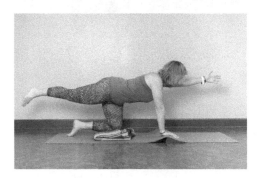

b: Cat-Cow

Start on the hands and knees with support under the knees and wrists as needed. Hands can also be placed into fists or on fingertips. Alternatively, the elbows can rest on yoga blocks to remove weight from the hands. You may experiment with bringing the knee toward the chest then lengthening the leg behind you or raising a leg, arm, or opposite leg and arm, being sure to keep the pelvis and shoulder girdle parallel with the floor. This sequence can also be done sitting in a chair, beginning in Seated *Tadasana*. For Cat, round the back, bringing the belly toward the spine and the whole spine into a C-shaped curve. For Cow, arch the back, opening the chest and front body. Sequence between these two poses in coordination with the breath, exhaling into Cat and inhaling into Cow.

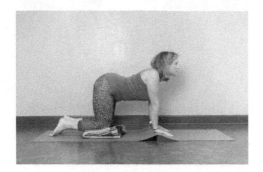 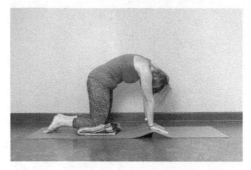

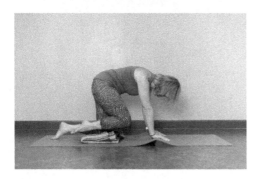 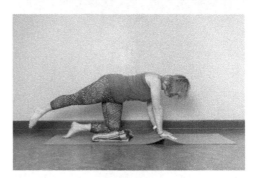

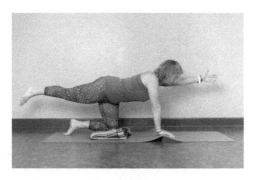 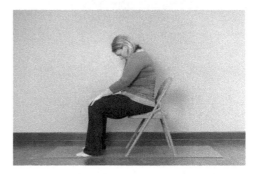

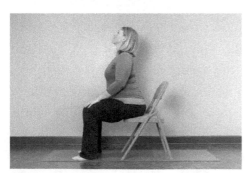

E: Seated Postures

a: Staff

Staff Pose is a seated posture with the legs extended and a long vertical spine. It can be done on the floor or seated in a chair with the legs resting on another chair. Hands may rest on the lap or beside the hips with whatever hand variation works for the wrists, keeping shoulders relaxed back and down. Props should be placed under the hips and knees as needed in order to allow for a long spine and greater comfort in the low back. Over time, small leg lifts may be added to this posture as quadriceps strength and hamstring flexibility improve. Simply engaging the thigh muscles is helpful, even if the leg doesn't move. Be sure to avoid leaning back, as a vertical spine is more important than the height of the leg.

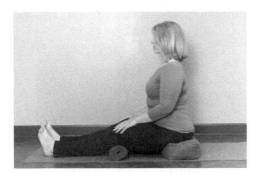
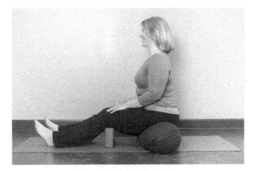

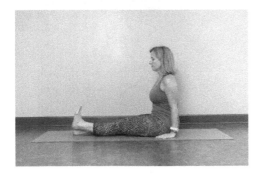

b: Seated Twist

Start in Staff pose, either on the floor or in a chair, perhaps sitting on a prop (blanket, pillow, bolster). On the floor, pull one knee in as if preparing for Head-to-Knee Pose. You might choose to leave the foot planted on the floor or lift and cross it over to the outside of the extended leg. In either case, imagine making a footprint on the floor. Drawing the foot in close to the body may help you sit up taller, as long as it feels okay for the hip and knee. Wrap the opposite arm around the bent knee, hugging it toward the body as you sit tall and keep sitz bones planted evenly on the floor. In a chair, you may choose to keep the feet firmly planted or cross one leg over the other. Sit up tall and begin to twist from the base of the spine toward the crossed leg, looking gently over shoulder.

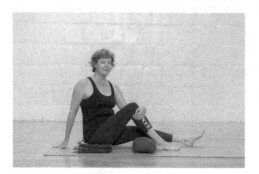

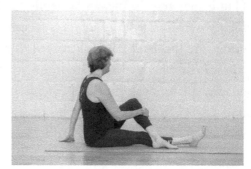

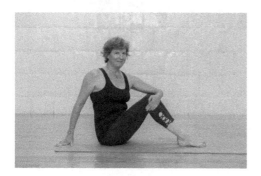

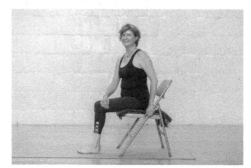

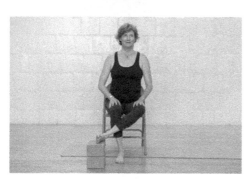

c: Tailor's Pose

Sit with knees bent out to the sides, soles of the feet touching. It is also an option to bring just one foot toward the groin and leave the other leg extended, either in front or to the side. Heels/ankles are encouraged in close to the body as possible, which may not be very far. Sit on a blanket, bolster, or block to help lengthen the spine and keep the torso upright. If uncomfortable, blocks can be placed under the knees for support. You may angle or roll forward, gazing past the feet to keep the neck long or tucking the chin.

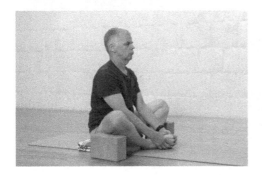 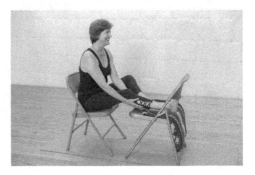

d: Centering Variations

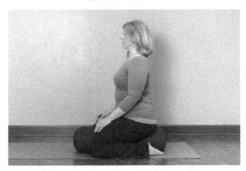 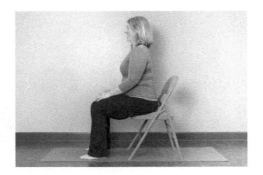

F: Forward-Bending Postures

a: Forward Fold

You might walk the feet toward the front from Downward Dog or come into Forward Fold from standing. When hinging at the hips, keep the spine long and avoid taking the arms forward, which adds pressure to the spine. You may want to use the support of a wall or chair, or walk the hands down the thighs as you lower. Be sure the knees stay soft, not locked, and that the weight remains distributed evenly across the feet without rolling in or out. If bending past vertical, the upper body can release and surrender into the pose. Hands may rest on blocks, you can hold opposite elbows, or just let the arms hang.

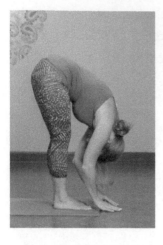
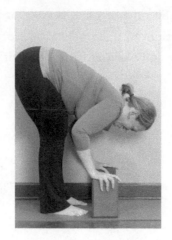
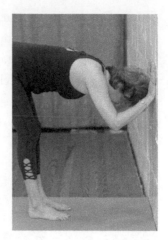
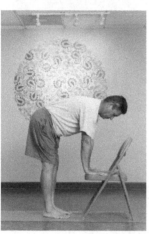
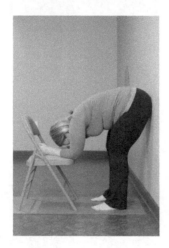
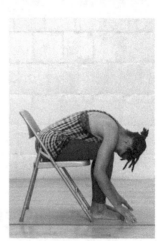

b: Head to Knee

Starting in Staff Pose on the floor or a chair, bend one knee toward the chest, planting the foot on the floor. Let the knee open out to the side with the sole of the foot touching the inside of the opposite leg (like in Tree). You may want some support, like a block or blanket, under the knee. Knee and toes of the straight leg point up toward the ceiling. Sitting up tall might be the full pose for some. If you have room to hinge forward, keep a long spine as you, walk the hands down the sides of the extended leg. Work to center the sternum over the thigh so that the shoulders are somewhat even. Taking a look at the elbows can assist with this. They should be the same distance from the floor. A strap can be wrapped under the sole of the foot, holding onto the strap with both hands or looping the arms through the strap. Keep a long spine unless folding to 45 degrees, at which point you can release forward and surrender.

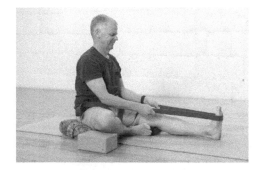
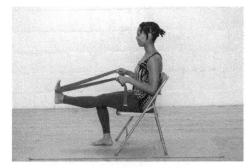
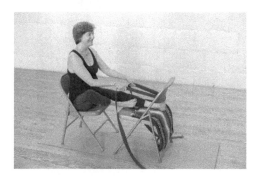
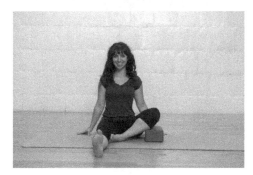
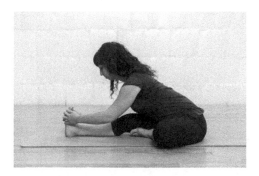

c: Seated Forward Fold

Start in Staff Pose on the floor or in a chair, perhaps sitting up on a prop (blanket, pillow, bolster) or supporting the knees if the hamstrings are tight. Lengthen the spine and begin to hinge forward from the hips. A strap can be wrapped under the soles of the feet, holding on with both hands to deepen the pose. Arms can extend actively alongside the legs or walk slowly down the legs and rest. Be sure to keep a long and active spine. If you are comfortably past 45 degrees, you may want to let the torso relax toward the legs, perhaps onto a bolster. If seated in a chair, be sure to stay stable and safe when folding forward.

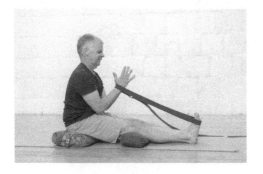
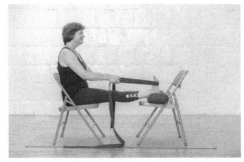
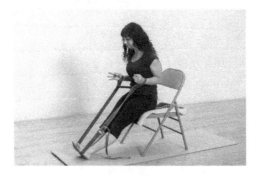
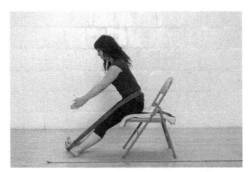
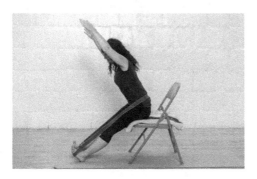
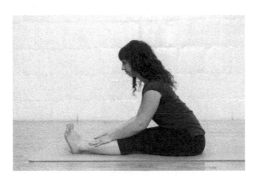

d: Downward Dog

From Table on the floor, you can tuck toes under and lift knees to downward dog or come up in a way that is more comfortable for the feet. It is fine if the heels don't touch, but be sure not to hold the heels up artificially. Let them drop toward the floor or into a prop such as a wedge or blanket. Hips reach toward the ceiling with the head relaxed and gaze is toward the toes. Knees are soft and not locked. If possible, palms press firmly into the mat, like trying to make a handprint. Any variations or props that were used in Table can be used here, too, in support of the hands and wrists. Downward Dog can be done with hands on a chair or wall for a smaller hip angle. It can also be done seated with the hands on the back of another chair, with arms extended, or with elbows on the knees. Note that the chair may be oriented so that you are working with the seat or the back of the chair. It is also an option to change orientation, sit on a chair, and create length from tailbone through top of head while supporting arms against thighs.

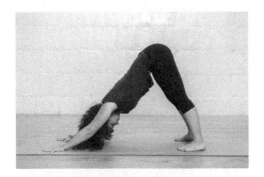
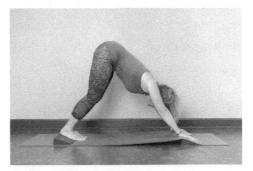

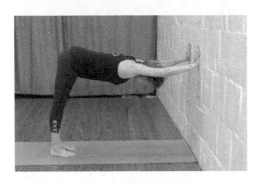
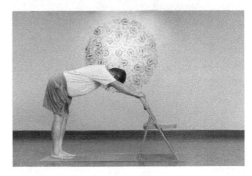

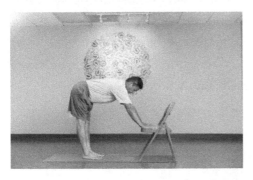
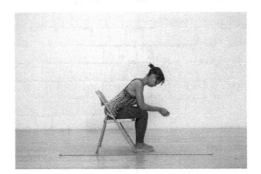

G: Backward-Bending Postures

a: Cobra

Lying prone with tops of the feet resting on the floor, palms are flat on the floor alongside the chest, elbows in close to the body. For those unable to place their palms on the floor, they can use fists or elbows. Head, neck, and chest are lifted off the floor. Gaze forward, keeping the feet and legs down. Upper-back muscles should be engaged so the arms are not used to execute the movement. Students can test this by trying to lift hands from the floor and maintain the pose. For more of a challenge, interlace fingers behind back to draw shoulder blades together (or hold opposite wrist).

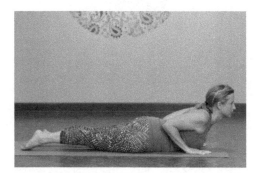 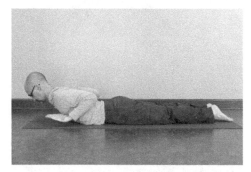

b: Sphinx

Sphinx can be used as an alternative to Cobra, especially for those with wrist or hand arthritis. The elbows are right under the shoulders so that the upper arm is perpendicular to the floor. Gently glide the shoulders away from the ears to broaden the chest. Abdominal muscles are engaged to protect the lumbar spine. The lower ribs and possibly the abdomen may be lifted off the floor. Placing a prop under the hips (pillow, folded blanket) can reduce pressure on the low back.

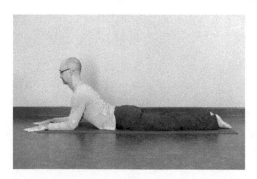 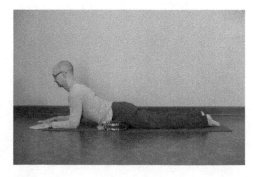

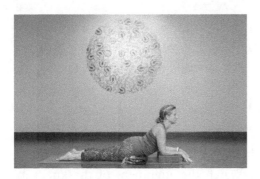

c: Locust

Begin lying on the abdomen, arms alongside the body. Rest the forehead on the floor or a folded blanket for a few breaths. Try rocking the body side to side, tucking the hands under the thighs, palms facing up. Some students may be able to tuck the elbows inside the hip bones. If neither of these positions is comfortable, the arms can be to the sides of the body. Having the palms face down may provide more stability. For half locust, lift one leg, keeping the hips level, forehead or chin can remain on the floor to support the cervical spine. Switch to the other leg. If you want to try Full Locust, bring both legs together and lift simultaneously. This is challenging and legs may not lift very high. Be sure to keep knees lengthened, since there is a tendency to bend the knees for greater height. Once again, it is not about the height of the pose, but the intention, muscle engagement, breath, and integrity of the alignment. Focus on engagement of the core muscles and be sure there is no aggravation of the low back or neck.

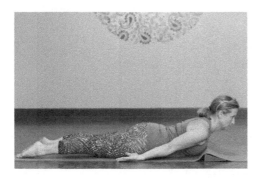

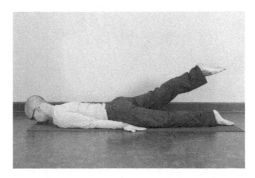

d: Bow

Many people will benefit from using a strap for this pose. Start by lying prone and bringing the forehead to the mat, so the cervical spine is long. Bend both knees, wrapping the strap around the front of both ankles. This may require some assistance, as it might be difficult for to reach. Alternatively, you can hold onto pant legs or feet or simply reach behind you. Lifting the head and pulling on the strap or feet, the whole body arches, shoulder blades drawing together while remaining strong through the front of the shoulders. Watch the alignment of the knees in comparison to hips and ankles—they should all be in one plane. If this stresses the spine, just lifting the head and holding the strap is enough, without arching the whole back.

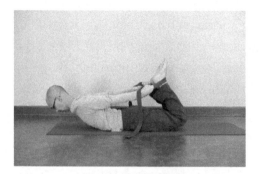 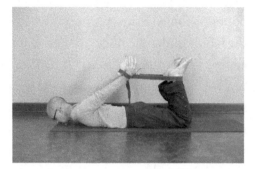

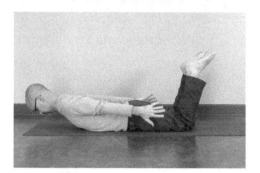

e: Bridge

To prepare for Bridge, lie on the back, soles of the feet placed on the floor, about one foot from the hips or whatever distance is comfortable for the knees. Feet should be hipbone-distance apart and knees pointing straight upward. Arms are extended alongside the body. Pressing into the feet, hips are lifted just slightly off of the floor. Some people may not have enough strength to lift the hips, which is fine.

Continue to engage the muscles as if they were going to lift, and eventually it will build more strength to facilitate a lift. It is important to continue breathing and not strain to accomplish the movement. There is a tendency for the knee positioning to be compromised, and for the angle of the feet to change during execution. Toes should point straight forward. If necessary, a strap can be used to keep the knees from opening outward, perhaps even with a block between the knees. For more of a challenge (or when doing several rounds), you can try reaching the hands for the heels, overhead (if the shoulders allow) and/or lift one leg at a time toward the ceiling. For a more restorative version of the pose, a prop can be placed under the sacrum, such as a block, cushion, or folded blanket.

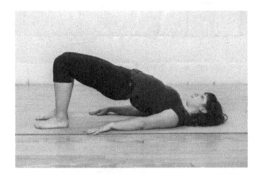
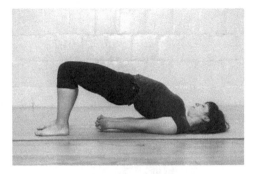
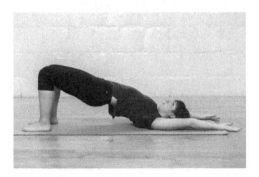
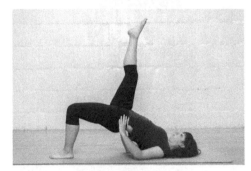

f: Camel

Start standing on the knees, possibly placing a blanket under the knees for support. Knees are hip-distance apart with the feet right behind the knees, tops of the feet resting on the mat or toes tucked under. Support under the knees or ankles may be needed. Fingers can be interlaced or hold onto the opposite wrist or a strap. Draw shoulder blades together and lift the gaze. With arthritis, it is important not to drop the head back, but to gently lift the eyes and open the throat. If comfortable, hands can be placed on a block between the feet, or to hold the heels. This can also be done in a chair, beginning in Seated *Tadasana*. Reach the arms around the back of the chair, holding onto the sides or back. Draw shoulder blades together and lift the gaze, opening the heart and throat. Feel an opening in the lungs and deepening of the breath.

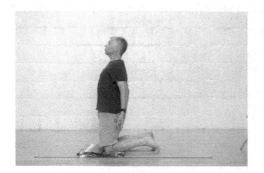
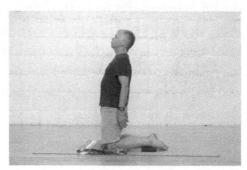

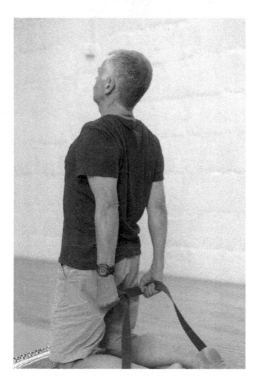
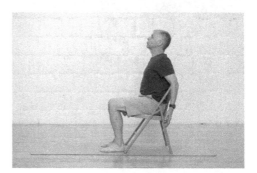

H: Lying Postures

a: Lying Extended Leg

Lying on back, pull one knee in toward chest, holding behind the knee instead of in front of the knee. Allow the extended leg to relax on the floor, with support under that knee as needed. Most students will want to use a strap, wrapping it under the sole of the foot to extend the leg upward toward the ceiling. The strap can be under any portion of the foot that feels comfortable (ball, heel, arch). You can alternatively hold the back of the leg as it extends, or even the fabric of loose pants. Instead of holding the two ends of the strap in each hand, you can also create a loop with the strap and feed the arms through with elbows bent, hands coming toward the torso. This may work better for those with arthritis in the hands. If not too much strain for the neck, the head can be lifted toward the knee, drawing the abdominal muscles in toward the spine. After lowering the head down, you can continue by bringing both ends of the strap (or the loop) into one hand on the side of the lifted leg. The other hand should be placed on the hip of the lower leg to keep it stable. The upper leg opens out to the side, being sure to keep both hips on the floor. The leg can remain in the air or be placed on a prop (chair, block, bolster). If the hips are stable, the other arm can be extended out to the side, with the head turning in that direction. Switching the strap to the other hand, you can then move into an extended-leg version of lying spinal twist.

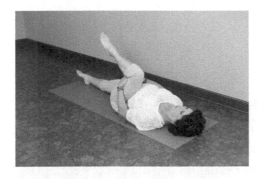
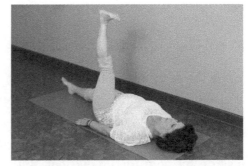
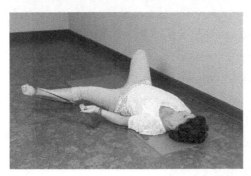
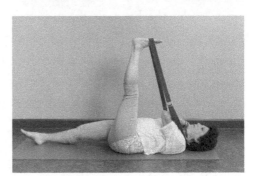

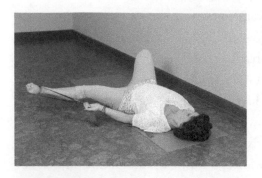
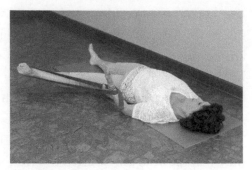
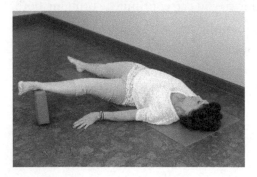

b: Lying Spinal Twist

Using the strap and continuing from lying extended leg pose, the leg can be brought across the body to the floor on the other side. For a gentler variation, bend the knee back into the body and let the bent knee cross toward the floor on the opposite side. To begin this pose on its own, lay supine, draw one knee in toward the torso and take it across the body toward the floor. With either variation (leg straight or bent), place props under the knee, thigh, and/or foot for support. The other arm can extend out to the side and the head might turn in that direction if it feels comfortable. Although there is some active stretching of the hamstrings when holding the strap or leg, the spinal twist is passive. The leg should be relaxed on the floor/props as the opposite shoulder reaches toward the floor. It is fine if the shoulder doesn't touch, and the hip of the top leg should be off the floor so the twist extends through the whole spine. For another variation, the spinal twist can occur after Bridge Pose, starting with both knees bent into the chest, dropping both knees over to one side. The arms are extended out to the sides if that works for the shoulders and the head turns away from the knees if possible. No strap is needed for this pose, but a block between the knees may be helpful. In any spinal twist, if it is too intense for arthritis in the spine, the legs can rest on a prop (block, chair, bolster, blanket) to decrease the intensity of the pose. If turning the head is bothersome, that step can be left out.

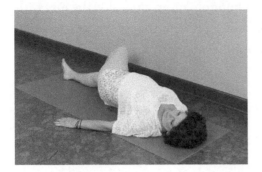 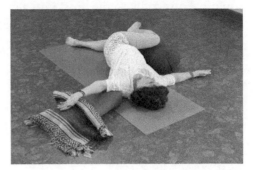

1: Standing Postures

a: Mountain

Mountain Pose can be done standing or seated. In either position, there should be a sense of grounding through the feet or the seat as well as a lengthening of the spine. In this pose, close your eyes and focus inward for a moment, scanning the body, noticing the movement of energy and the body's alignment. Fell the knees over the ankles, the shoulders over the hips. Follow a few deep breaths and notice the state of the body and mind. This pose can be used throughout the day as a way to check in and become mindful. It can also be used as a pause between poses in a yoga practice to re-center and observe any changes.

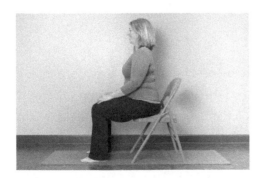 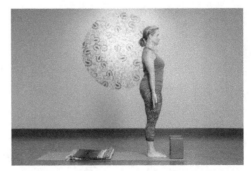

b: Warrior I

From *Tadasana*, step the front foot back into a lunge and rotate the back leg out slightly, so the outside of the foot can press into the floor. If this is not accessible, it is fine to stay up on the ball of the back foot or place a prop under the heel. If the back leg is not rotated in enough, you will be unable to bring both hips square. Arms come to the hips, into a cactus position, or up alongside the ears with shoulders relaxed and fingers extended. Shoulders should be aligned back over the hips with the gaze straight ahead. A deep bend in the front knee should not bring the knee past the ankle.

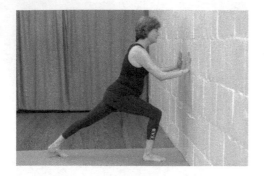
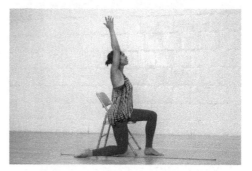
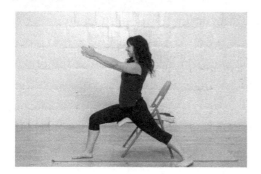
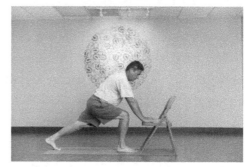

c: Warrior II

This is the first standing pose to be introduced and feels awkward to many students at the beginning. There are a lot of postural considerations, so take your time experimenting with variations. The stance should be wider than most would imagine. After stepping wide on the mat, hold the arms straight out, with wrists and shoulders in one line. Look at the feet to ensure they are positioned under the palms. You may have to step wider to accomplish this, which will be important for knee alignment later in the pose. Toes on the front foot turn 90 degrees to face front, and toes on the back foot turn 45 degrees to face the corner. Many will not turn this back foot in enough, which will hinder the ability to orient the hips properly. If you have limitations in the ankle, due to fused bones, deformity, or joint pain, put a wedge or block under the back heel.

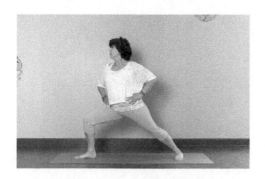

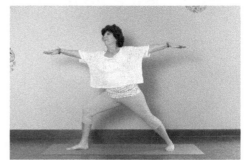

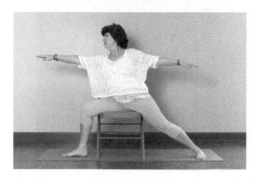

d: Reverse Warrior

From the Warrior II stance, the back hand comes to rest on the outside of the back leg. It is not important how far down the leg this is. The hand can also rest on the back hip, if that is more comfortable. The front arm reaches overhead in an arc, straight up, or in cactus. The front hand can also rest on the shoulder. Gaze is traditionally up into the palm, but take care to protect the neck. It is fine to look forward, if that feels better. Bend the knee deeply, as in Warrior I or II, being sure that the knee does not extend past the ankle and that weight is distributed evenly through the front foot. A wedge or other prop can be placed under the back heel or outside edge of the foot as needed.

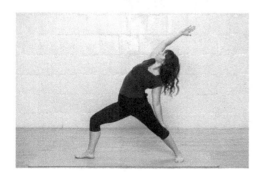

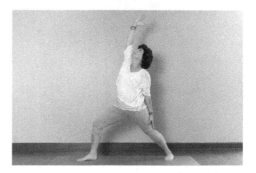

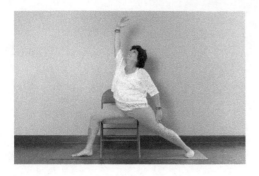

J: Side-Bending Postures

a: Triangle

Begin in the same stance as Warrior II, with the front knee straightened but not locked. Stand up tall with arms extended to the sides and shift the torso forward toward the front leg, reaching forward with the front arm. From there, begin tilting the torso sideways so that the hand naturally reaches a resting place on your leg, a block, or a chair. Make sure you are not reaching too far down and compromising the alignment of the torso; keep one shoulder stacked over the other. Think about opening the front of that upper shoulder with the arm reaching toward the ceiling. The hand can also be placed on the upper hip, with the elbow reaching upward. The gaze is traditionally up toward the open palm but can be straight ahead or down for more comfort in the neck.

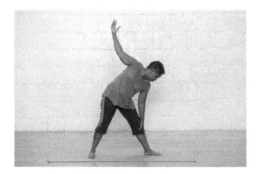
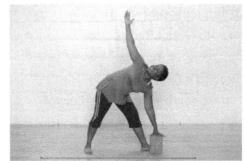

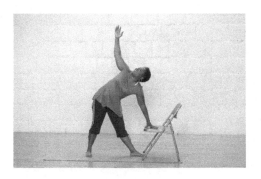
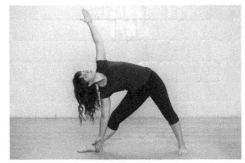

b: Side Angle

Starting in Warrior II, bring the front elbow to rest on the bent knee. Be sure that the knee is stacked over the ankle and not past. To go deeper, you might try lowering that hand to a block, keeping one shoulder stacked over the other. The other arm can extend alongside body, into cactus, or up alongside the ear. You can also bring the hand to rest on the upper hip. The goal is one continuous diagonal line from the back foot to the extended arm or crown of the head. You can gaze past the extended fingers, past the upper shoulder, or straight ahead. Watch for tension or condensing in the lower shoulder as you lean into the supporting elbow. The hips and shoulders should be in one plane, as though laying against a wall. Release any tension in the hand and fingers of the extended arm. Focus on a healthy alignment rather than trying to achieve a certain shape or depth in the pose.

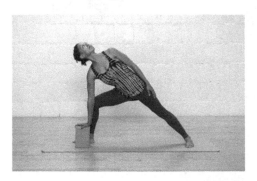
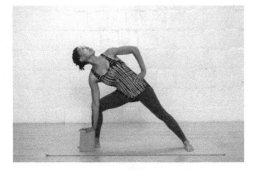

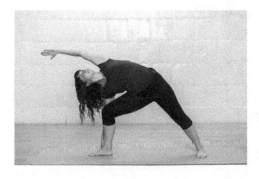

K: Balancing Postures

a: Tree

Standing on both feet, perhaps with the support of a chair or wall for balance, begin to shift the weight toward the left foot, coming to the ball of the foot on the right side. Rotate the right leg out from the hip and bring the right foot close to the left ankle. You can stay here or try bringing the right foot to rest on the inside of the left ankle. Be sure toes point straight down, not forward. You might want to try sliding the right foot up to the left calf, or even using the right hand to bring the right foot up to the left thigh. Be sure to avoid putting the foot directly on the knee. The right leg acts like a buttress for a building to keep you steady, with pressure of foot and leg against each other creating resistance to maintain the pose. Keep length in the left-side body without sinking into the left hip. Hands can be on the hips, at the heart, in cactus, or overhead. Keep shoulders relaxing down. If you are holding onto the foot, be sure not to hunch upper body forward, but to keep vertical spine. The gaze is up and out, on a focal point of your choice. Breathe deeply and repeat on the other side.

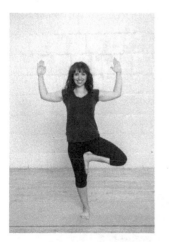
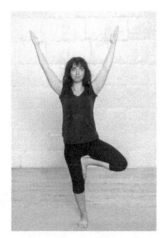
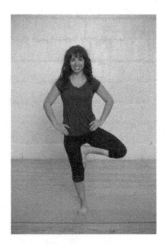

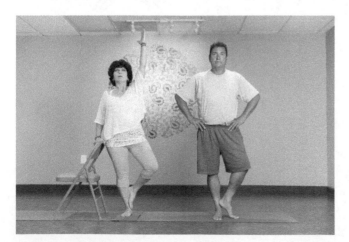

b: Eagle

One knee crosses over the other, bringing them as close as possible, which is easier with a deep bend in knees and hips or seated in a chair. It can also be done against a wall for stability and support. For those with arthritis in hips, knees, ankles, or feet, it is not necessary to try bringing the foot around the back of the calf, as is done traditionally. It may be more comfortable to rest the foot on a block or other prop. The elbows cross in the opposite manner. It is fine if the elbows don't touch. More important is the idea of opposing twists. The lower body twists and crosses in one direction, while the upper body twists and crosses in the other direction, bringing the body back to center. Whether or not the palms are touching, fingers should be elongated and pointed upward, aiming to keep the eyes between the hands or the hands between the eyes.

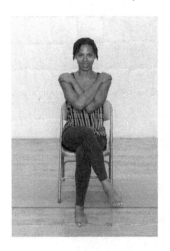 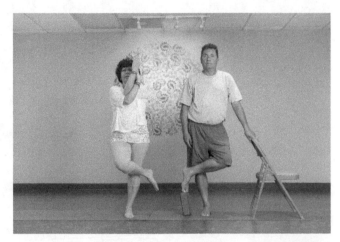

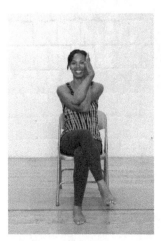 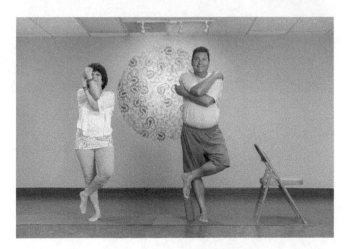

c: Extended Leg

This may be done with a strap, or by holding the outside of the knee. It can be a balancing pose near the wall or can build strength and flexibility when seated in a chair. It is far more important to maintain a long, healthy spine than to reach the toe. The other hand can be placed on the hip or extended overhead. From this position, the leg can be brought out to one side, ensuring that the hip does not lift or internally rotate. It is also important to keep the other hip aligned with knee and ankle, without leaning to the outside of the supporting foot. If feeling stable, you can take the other arm out to the side and/or turn the head to look the other way.

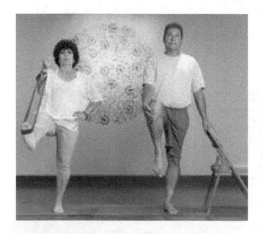 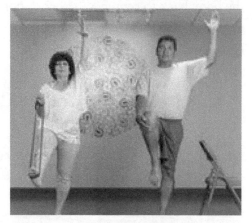

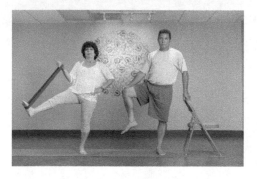 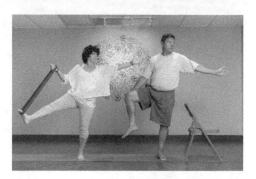

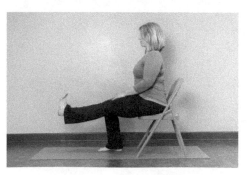 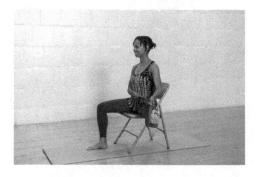

d: King Dancer

Most students will want to use a strap or chair for this pose. To use a strap, begin standing by the wall or a chair for support and wrap the strap around the front of the ankle, holding onto it with one hand or looping it over the same shoulder. Alternatively, place the foot or knee on a chair behind you. Hip/knee/ankle should be in one plane (so the knee is not torqued) and hips are square to the front. If feeling stable, the other arm can be raised overhead or to a cactus position. For greater challenge, the pose can be tipped forward with one line from fingertips to knee. There is a tendency for the angle of the hip to decrease or the back to round when extending forward. It is more important to keep a long spine than to tip forward. The supporting knee should be soft, with weight evenly distributed on the whole foot.

A seated version of the pose begins in Seated *Tadasana*, with one knee lowering to the side of the chair. Be sure to avoid a pulling sensation in the front of the knee, so the stretch is felt more in the middle of the thigh and/or hip flexors.

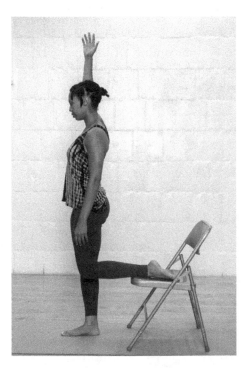
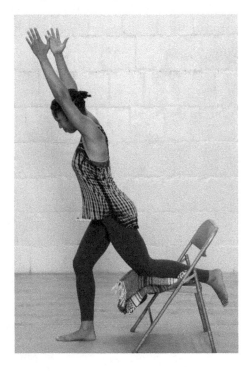

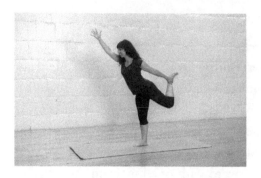

e: Half-Moon

This is a fairly advanced pose and is not introduced until late in the session, perhaps moving from a standing pose or other balance. I recommend using a block (at any height) or a chair to support the pose without reaching for the floor. There is an intention toward creating one line from head to the heel of the extended leg. The other hand can be on the hip or reaching toward the ceiling within the limits of comfort for the shoulder. Gaze can be upward toward an extended arm, straight forward, or down toward the floor, depending on the comfort of the neck. This is best done against a wall at first, lying back against the wall to feel the expansiveness of the pose. It can then be replicated just an inch away from the wall to challenge balance, if desired.

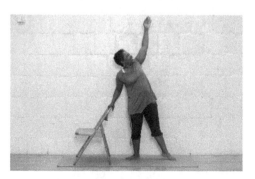 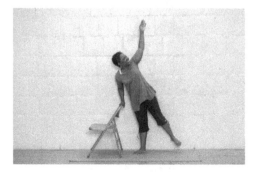

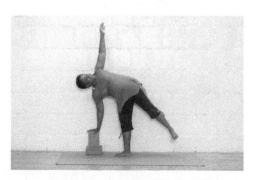 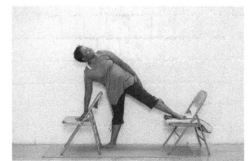

f: Warrior III

You may want to begin preparations for Warrior III at a chair or wall for support. This is a challenging pose, but it can be modified for broader accessibility. Begin by shifting weight into the left foot and extending the right foot back so that just the toes are touching the floor behind you. You can try lifting the right hand off of the chair/wall and extending it overhead or to cactus position. This may be your Warrior III. Consider a long line of energy extending from the left leg to the right arm and maintain the alignment of that line. If you like, you can begin lifting the left toes and tipping the torso forward. It is more important to maintain the line from fingertips to the heel of the extended leg than it is to tip forward. In fact, you might stay relatively upright, which is fine. Be sure that as you go deeper into the pose, the supporting knee remains soft, with weight distributed throughout the whole foot. Gaze can be down or straight ahead. Gently return to *Tadasana* and repeat on the other side.

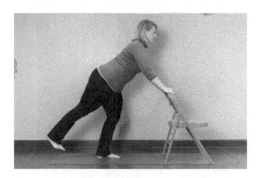 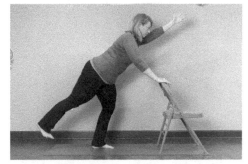

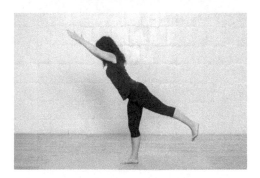

L: *Vinyasas*

a: *Straddle*

Start with legs as wide as they would be for Warrior II, but with toes both pointing straight ahead. Take your arms out to the sides for reference and consider bringing the feet as wide as the hands. Internally rotate the legs slightly (heels out, toes in). Hands are placed on the hips, with shoulder blades drawn together and down. Fold forward at the hips, trying not to lean back into the heels. If you feel unstable with the hands on the hips, they can be placed on floor, block, or chair. Bring torso over one leg, holding onto that leg with both hands (or keeping one hand on floor/block/ chair for support), keeping the hips from shifting to the opposite side. Shift to the other side. Come back to center. You can try bringing the arms around the back and hold a strap or opposite wrist. Release arms slowly to the sides. Walk legs in to shoulder distance apart, bend the knees and lengthen the spine up to Mountain.

This can also be done seated in a chair. Begin in Seated *Tadasana* and take the feet wide with knees over ankles. Shift the torso over one thigh and then the other before coming to center. For safety, take the hands to a prop such as blocks or another chair. Place hands on thighs and press up to vertical, returning to Seated *Tadasana*.

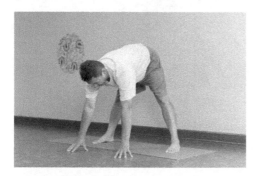
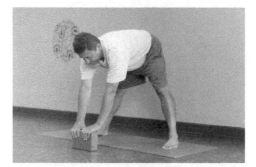

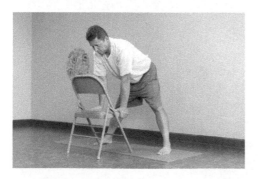
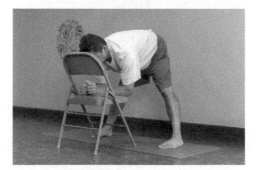

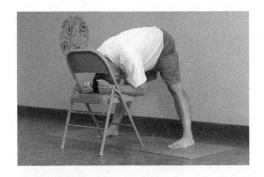

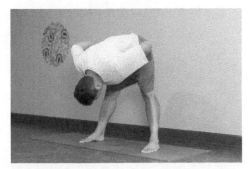

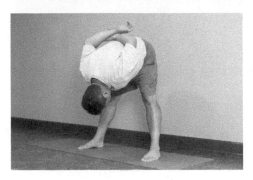

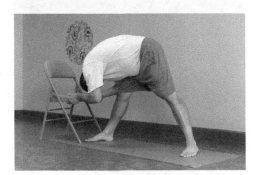

b: Standing Sun Salutations

Sun Salutation is a fluid sequence and while each step may take time in the beginning, eventually you will move through the poses without stopping. For starters, go through each pose slowly to ensure you have proper alignment and understanding in each before moving on. You may find that it is a challenge just to move through the sequence once. Once it becomes more comfortable, you may want to move through a few rounds as a warm-up to your practice, as a way to greet the day, or as a break from sedentary work.

1. Stand in Mountain. Bring the palms together in front of the heart.

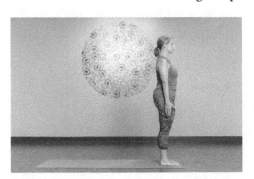

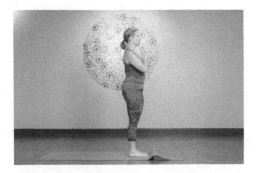

2. Arch back—Just the upper body from beneath the shoulder blades. Hips should remain stable to protect lower back.

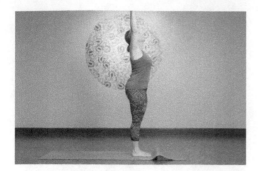

3. Forward Fold—Hinge at the hips with long spine and soft knees. Consider resting hands on blocks or other prop.

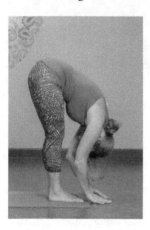

4. Lunge—Step back with left foot in the first round and right in the second round, etc. Be sure the front knee does not bend past the ankle. Chest should be open to the front with the eyes up and out. The back leg should be far enough back that there is a stretch in the hip flexors on that side. The back knee can be on or off the floor. You may want a blanket under the knee for cushioning. Hands should be on either side of the front foot, perhaps on fingertips or blocks.

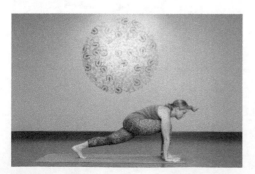 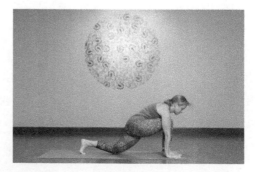

5. Downward Dog (see page 284).

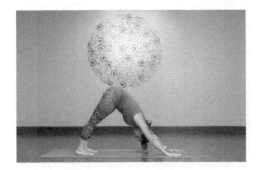 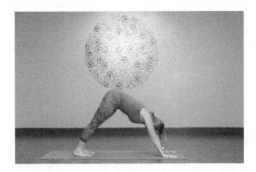

6. Table to Prone—Lower knees to the floor and then come to lying on the abdomen. No weight should be in the hands. Try to avoid lowering to the elbows and sliding legs back to get hips down. Instead, hands and knees stay where they are and the torso moves forward to the floor (hands on either side of the chest). Use hand variations as needed (fists, blocks, wedge).

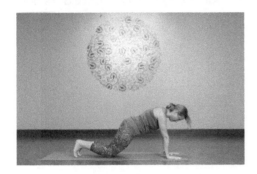

7. Cobra (see page 286).

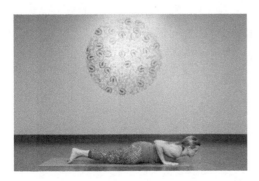 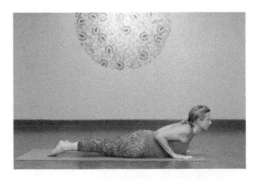

8. Downward Dog (see page 284).

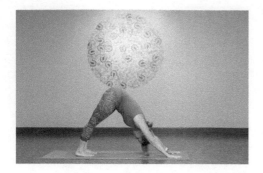 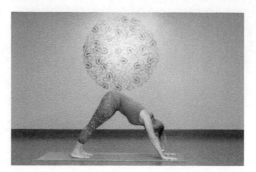

9. Lunge (other leg)—Step forward between hands. This is a challenging transition. You might want to step forward halfway, lower the other knee, and use your arm to bring the foot all the way through. You can also lower to both knees before stepping forward. Putting blocks at the front of the mat will make this easier. Be sure to step all the way forward, so the knee does not go past the ankle in the lunge.

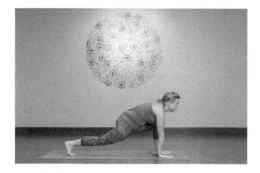

10. Forward Fold—Step back leg forward to meet front leg.

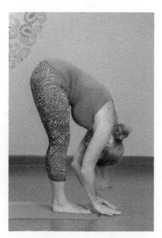

11. Arch back—Inhale arms up and elongate the front of the body.

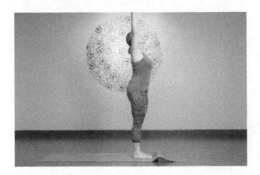

12. Mountain—Palms draw in to the heart and lower down. If repeating the sequence, go right from hands at the heart into arch again for the next round.

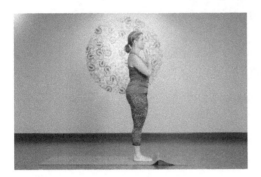

c: Wall-Assisted Sun Salutation

1. Begin in *Tadasana*, facing the wall, with about a 2-foot distance between your stance and the wall. You may need to adjust that distance according to your torso and limb lengths.

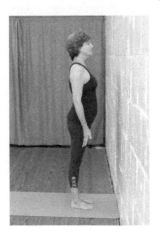

2. Reach the arms out to the side and up overhead on an inhale, arching slightly back from the ribcage.

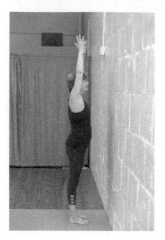 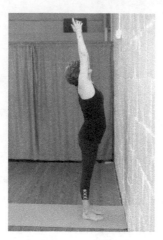

3. Hinge forward at the hips, walking the hands slowly down the wall with a long spine. You can choose to stop when the spine is horizontal with the floor or continue lowering further into Forward Fold.

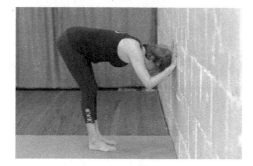

4. From here, bring the palms, fists, or fingertips to the wall and step the left foot back into a lunge, being sure that the front knee does not extend past the front ankle. If this occurs, step the back foot further back to allow for a deeper lunge.

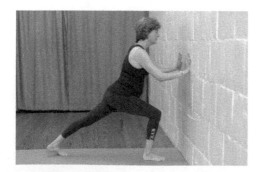

5. From the lunge, step the right foot back to meet the left for a modified Downward Dog. Hips reach back away from the wall with a long, horizontal spine.

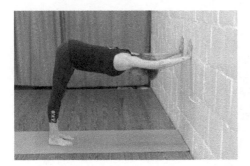

6. Walk in a bit closer to the wall, bringing the hips toward the wall and take a gentle backbend by opening the heart and throat. The closer you step to the wall, the gentler this modified Cobra Pose will be. Palms, fingertips, or fists rest on the wall with elbows close in to the body and core engaged to support the lower back.

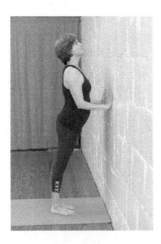

7. Step the left foot forward into a lunge on the other side and then bring the back foot in to meet the front foot.

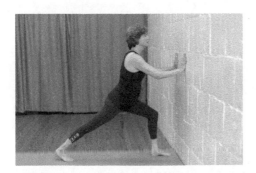

8. Reach the arms up overhead (to whatever extent is comfortable) with a gentle arch back and bring the hands back to the heart, returning to *Tadasana*.

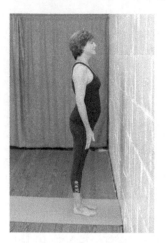 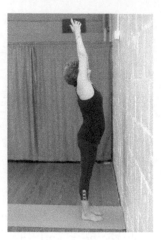

9. Repeat another round with the right foot, stepping forward and back. Continue as many repetitions as feels good and appropriate for you today.

d: Sun Salutations with a Chair

1. Begin standing in *Tadasana* behind the chair, which is placed securely on a yoga mat. For a gentler version of the sequence, face the chair back toward you. For more intensity, turn the chair seat toward you.

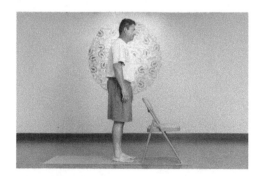

2. Bring hands to the heart in whatever orientation is comfortable for the hands and wrists.

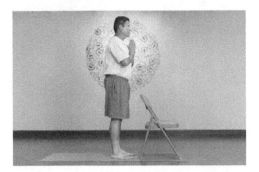

3. Reach the arms upward, opening the heart and throat, bending gently backward from the ribcage upward while the rest of the body remains tall and stable.

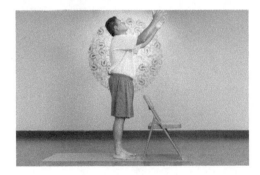

4. Hinge at the hips and fold over the chair, bringing the hands to rest on the chair. Be sure that the knees are soft and not locked. Maintain a long spine with space between the vertebrae.

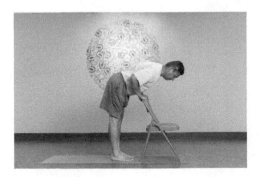

5. Step the left foot back into a lunge. You may want to place a wedge under the back heel for support. Be sure to step back far enough that the front knee does not bend past the ankle.

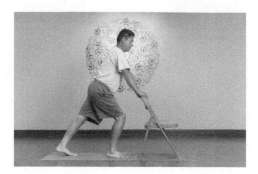

6. Step the right foot back to meet the left and reach the hips back into a modified Downward Dog, holding onto the chair and finding length in the spine.

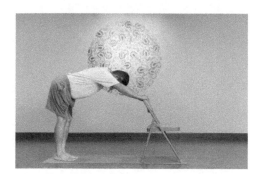

7. Reach the hips forward toward the chair for a modified Cobra Pose. You may want to step closer to the chair for Cobra. The closer you are to the chair, the less weight the hands must support.

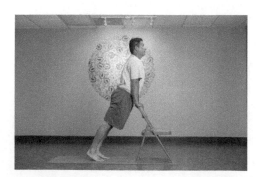

8. From Cobra, press back into Downward Dog again.

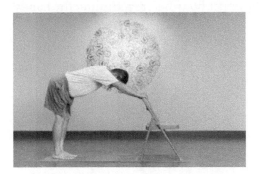

9. Step the right foot forward into a lunge on the other side, again being sure that the knee does not go past the ankle.

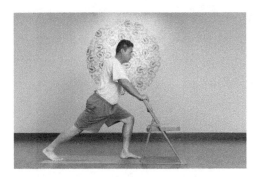

10. Step the back foot forward and fold over the chair.

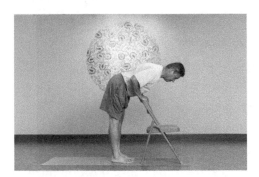

11. Bend the knees and use the support of the chair to come back up, reaching up and gently back into an arch of the upper body before returning the hands to the heart.

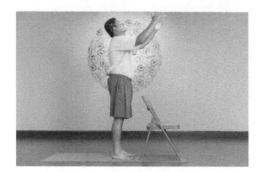 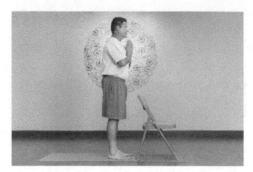

12. Repeat the sequence on the other side, with the right leg reaching back into the lunge. Finish the sequence with *Tadasana* and reflect on any changes in the body. Notice differences in energy, breath, thoughts, and sensations. You may choose to use this sequence to greet the day, to begin your yoga practice, or as an occasional break from sedentary work.

M: Relaxation

a: Savasana

Savasana is traditionally done lying on the back without any propping. For a supported *Savasana*, you can experiment with what will be most comfortable, relaxing and sustainable for the duration of the progressive relaxation. Because *Savasana* lasts several minutes and the focus should be on restoration and relaxation, it is important to find a position without strain. You may want to put a rolled blanket under the knees, rest the lower legs on a chair, place a narrowly folded blanket along the spine, support the lumbar region, or place something under the head. These are a few examples, but take your time and make adjustments until you feel satisfied with the position. Even then, it is okay to change position during *Savasana* if it is no longer comfortable or is hindering relaxation.

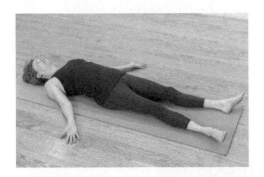

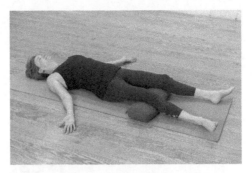

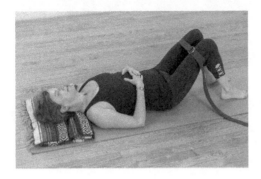

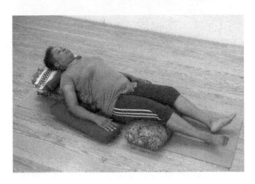

Resources

Books

Yoga Sutras of Patanjali, Swami Satchidananda (trans.)

The Bhagavad Gita, Ecknath Easwaran (trans.)

Science of Breath, Swami Rama

Yoga Therapy for Stress and Anxiety, Robert Butera, Erin Byron, and Staffan Elgelid

Out of Joint, Mary Felstiner

Principles and Practices of Yoga in Healthcare, Sat Bir Singh Khalsa, Lorenzo Cohen, Timothy McCall, and Shirley Telles (eds)

Yoga, the Body, and Embodied Social Change, Jen Aubrecht

Yoga Therapy: A Personalized Approach to Your Active Lifestyle, Kristen Butera and Staffan Elgelid

Body Mindful, Robert Butera and Jennifer Kreatsoulas

Anatomy of Movement, Blandine Calais-Germain

Yoga and Science in Pain Care: Treating the Person in Pain, Shelly Prosko, Neil Pearson, and Marlysa Sullivan.

The Roll Model, Jill Miller

Meditation for Your Life, Robert Butera

Waking: A Memoir of Trauma and Transcendence, Matthew Sanford

Man's Search for Meaning, Victor Frankl

Yoga and the Quest for the True Self, Stephen Cope

Devotions, Mary Oliver

Yoga for the Creative Soul, Erin Byron

A Resilient Life, Kat Elton

The Power of One, Bryce Courtenay

The Secret Garden, Frances Hodgson Burnett (Reread it with fresh eyes)

A Mindful Nation, Tim Ryan (for Americans in need of hope and inspiration)

The Jew in the Lotus (for anyone curious about this common convergence of traditions)

Videos

Arthritis-Friendly Yoga, Arthritis Foundation (with Dr. Steffany Moonaz)

Yoga for the Rest of Us, Peggy Cappy

SmartCore Training, Staffan Elgelid

Online Resources

Yoga for Arthritis website. http://arthritis.yoga

Yoga for Arthritis—The Evidence and the Promise. https://www.yogauonline.com/yogau-product/4386

The Science Sutras. https://www.thesciencesutras.com

Creaky Joints. https://creakyjoints.org

Dianne Bondy. www.yogasteya.com

Yogamate. www.yogamate.org

Events and Trainings

Symposium on Yoga Therapy and Research (SYTAR)

www.iayt.org/?page=ConferenceLanding

Accessible Yoga Conferences. http://accessibleyoga.org

Yoga for Arthritis Teacher Trainings. https://arthritis.yoga/events

Comprehensive Yoga Therapy Training. www.yogalifeinstitute.com/teacher-training/yoga-therapy-training

Programs at Yogaville. https://www.yogaville.org

Yoga for Arthritis e-course. https://yogainternational.com/ecourse/yoga-for-arthritis

Arthritic Knees and Yoga. https://yogainternational.com/ecourse/arthritic-knees-yoga

Maryland University of Integrative Health. http://muih.edu/academics/masters-degrees/master-yoga-therapy

Anatomy and Yoga Therapy Conference. https://yogainternational.com/ecourse/anatomy-and-yoga-therapy-conference

Research

International Journal of Yoga Therapy. www.iayt.org/?page=AboutIJYT

Journal of Complementary and Alternative Medicine

Arthritis Care and Research

Explore: The Journal of Science and Healing. http://www.explorejournal.com/

ResearchGate. https://www.researchgate.net/profile/Steffany_Moonaz

Steffany Moonaz's Dissertation. https://pqdtopen.proquest.com/doc/375396720.html?FMT=ABS

Endnotes

Chapter 1

1. Barbour, K.E. *et al.* (2006) "Prevalence of Severe Joint Pain Among Adults with Doctor Diagnosed Arthritis—United States, 2002–2014." *MMWR.* 65, 1052–6.
2. European League Against Rheumatism. "Questions and Answers on Rheumatic Disease." Accessed October 26, 2017 at https://www.eular.org/myUploadData/files/Q-and-A-on-RMDs.pdf
3. Lawrence, R.C. *et al.* (2008) "Estimates of the Prevalence of Arthritis and Other Rheumatic Conditions in the United States: Part II." *Arthritis Rheum.* 58, 26–35.
4. Barbour, K.E. *et al.* (2017) "Vital Signs: Prevalence of Doctor-Diagnosed Arthritis and Arthritis-Attributable Activity Limitation—United States, 2013–2015." *MMWR.* 66, 9, 246–53.
5. Deane, K.D. *et al.* (2009) "Identification of Undiagnosed Inflammatory Arthritis in a Community Health-Fair Screen." *Arthritis Rheum.* 61, 12, 1642–9.
6. Hootman, J.M. *et al.* (2016) "Updated Projected Prevalence of Self-Reported Doctor-Diagnosed Arthritis and Arthritis-Attributable Activity Limitation Among US Adults, 2015–2040." *Arthritis Rheumatology.* 68, 7, 1582–7.
7. Barbour, K.E. *et al.* (2013) "Prevalence of Doctor-Diagnosed Arthritis and Arthritis-Attributable Activity Limitation—United States, 2010–2012." *MMWR.* 62, 44, 869–73.
8. Fernandes, L. *et al.* (2013) "EULAR Recommendations for the Non-Pharmacological Core Management of Hip and Knee Osteoarthritis." *Ann Rheum Dis.* 72, 7, 1125–35.
9. World Health Organization. (2001) "Department of Economic and Social Affairs World Population Ageing: 1950–2050." Accessed May 23, 2018 at www.un.org/esa/population/publications/worldageing19502050
10. Weinstein, S.I., Yelin, E.H., and Watkins-Castillo, S.I. (2014) "The Burden of Musculoskeletal Diseases (BMUS) in the United States, Fourth Edition." *The Big Picture.* Accessed May 23, 2018 at www.boneandjointburden.org/2014-report/i0/big-picture
11. Vollenhoven, R.F.V. (2009) "Sex Differences in Rheumatoid Arthritis: More Than Meets the Eye." *BMC Med.* 7, 12.
12. Cisternas, M.G. *et al.* (2015) "Alternative Methods for Defining Osteoarthritis and the Impact on Estimating Prevalence in a U.S. Population-Based Survey." *Arthritis Care Res (Hoboken).* 68, 5, 574–80.
13. World Health Organization. (2013) "Priority Medicines for Europe and the World Update Report." Accessed May 23, 2018 at www.who.int/medicines/areas/priority_medicines/Ch6_12Osteo.pdf

14. Hunter, D.J., Neogi, T., and Hochberg, M.C. (2011) "Quality of Osteoarthritis Management and the Need for Reform in the U.S." *Arthritis Care Res.* 63, 1, 31–8.

15. Mueller, M.B. and Tuan, R.S. (2011) "Anabolic/Catabolic Balance in Pathogenesis of Osteoarthritis: Identifying Molecular Targets." *PM R.* 3, 6 Suppl 1, S3–11.

16. Breedveld, F.C. (2004) "Osteoarthritis—The Impact of a Serious Disease." *Rheumatology*, 43, 1, i4–i8.

17. Sale, J.E.M, Gignac, M., and Hawker, G. (2008) "The Relationship Between Disease Symptoms, Life Events, Coping and Treatment, and Depression among Older Adults with Osteoarthritis." *Journal of Rheumatology.* 35, 2, 335–42.

18. Roubenoff, R.A. *et al.* (1994) "Rheumatoid Cachexia: Cytokine-Driven Hypermetabolism Accompanying Reduced Body Cell Mass in Chronic Inflammation." *J Clin Invest.* 93, 6, 2379–86.

19. Roubenoff, R. *et al.* (1992) "Rheumatoid Cachexia: Depletion of Lean Body Mass in Rheumatoid Arthritis: Possible Association with Tumor Necrosis Factor." *J Rheumatol.* 19, 10, 1505–10.

20. Taylor, P.C. *et al.* (2016) "A Structured Literature Review of the Burden of Illness and Unmet Needs in Patients with Rheumatoid Arthritis: A Current Perspective." *Rheumatology International.* 36, 5, 685–95.

21. Engel, Y.G.L. (1980) "The Clinical Application of the Biopsychosocial Model." *Am J Psychiatry*, 137, 5, 535–44.

22. Moonaz, S.H. *et al.* (2015) "Yoga in Sedentary Adults with Arthritis: Effects of a Randomized Controlled Pragmatic Trial." *J Rheumatol.* 42, 7, 1194–202.

23. *Ibid.*

24. Cramer, H. *et al.* (2015) "The Safety of Yoga: A Systematic Review and Meta-Analysis of Randomized Controlled Trials." *Am J Epidemiol.* 182, 4, 281–93.

25. Saper, R.B. *et al.* (2017) "Yoga, Physical Therapy, or Education for Chronic Low Back Pain: A Randomized Noninferiority Trial." *Ann Intern Med.* 167, 2, 85–94.

26. Jeter, P.E. *et al.* (2015) "Yoga as a Therapeutic Intervention: A Bibliometric Analysis of Published Research Studies from 1967 to 2013." *J Altern Complement Med.* 21, 10, 586–92.

27. Sullivan, M.B. *et al.* (2018) "Toward an Explanatory Framework for Yoga Therapy Informed by Philosophical and Ethical Perspectives." *Altern Ther Health Med.* 24, 1, 38–47.

28. Bolen, J. *et al.* (2010) "Differences in the Prevalence and Impact of Arthritis among Racial/Ethnic Groups in the United States, National Health Interview Survey, 2002, 2003, and 2006." *Prev Chronic Dis.* 7, 3, A64.

29. Lavernia, C.J. *et al.* (2011) "Ethnic and Racial Factors Influencing Wellbeing, Perceived Pain, and Physical Function after Primary Total Joint Arthroplasty." *Clin Orthop Relat Res.* 469, 7, 1838–45.

30. Greenberg, J.D. *et al.* (2013) "Racial and Ethnic Disparities in Disease Activity in Patients with Rheumatoid Arthritis." *Am J Med.* 126, 12, 1089–98.

31. Middleton, K.R. *et al.* (2018) "Feasibility and Assessment of Outcome Measures for Yoga as Self-Care for Minorities with Arthritis: A Pilot Study." *Pilot Feasibility Stud.* 4, 53; Middleton, K.R. et al. (2017) "A Qualitative Approach Exploring the Acceptability of Yoga for Minorities Living with Arthritis: 'Where Are the People Who Look Like Me?'" *Complementary Therapies in Medicine.* 31, 82–9; Middleton, K.R. *et al.* (2013) "Yoga Research and Spirituality: A Case Study Discussion." *Int J Yoga Therap.* 25, 1, 33–5; Middleton, K.R. *et al.* (2013) "Yoga and Physical Rehabilitation Medicine: A Research Partnership in Integrative Care." *J Yoga Phys Ther.* 3, 4, 149; Middleton, K.R. *et al.* (2013) "A Pilot Study of Yoga as Self-Care for Arthritis in Minority Communities." *Health Qual Life Outcomes.* 11, 55.

32. Arthritis Foundation. (2013) "Arthritis Foundation Launches Public Awareness Campaign in Conjunction with Arthritis Month this May." Accessed October 26, 2017 at www.prnewswire.

com/news-releases/arthritis-foundation-launches-public-awareness-campaign-in-conjunction-with-arthritis-month-this-may-205566761.html

33. Do You Yoga. (2017) "13 Organizations at the Forefront of Accessible Yoga." Accessed October 26, 2017 at www.doyouyoga.com/13-organizations-at-the-forefront-of-accessible-yoga-20750. See http://accessibleyoga.org

Chapter 2

34. Matcham, F. *et al.* (2014) "The Impact of Rheumatoid Arthritis on Quality-of-Life Assessed Using the SF-36: A Systematic Review and Meta-Analysis." *Seminars in Arthritis and Rheumatism.* 44, 2, 123–30.

35. For options, check out our video at www.youtube.com/watch?v=KXraelYVN0A

36. Engel, G.L. (1977) "The Need for a New Model of Medical Science: A Challenge for Biomedicine." *Science.* 196, 4286, 129–36.

37. Brown, J.L. *et al.* (2003) "Social Support and Experimental Pain." *Psychosomatic Medicine.* 65, 2, 276–83.

38. Rupp, I. *et al.* (2006) "Disability and Health-Related Quality of Life among Patients with Rheumatoid Arthritis: Association with Radiographic Joint Damage, Disease Activity, Pain, and Depressive Symptoms." *Scand J Rheumatol.* 35, 175–81.

Chapter 4

39. "Guidelines for the Management of Rheumatoid Arthritis: 2002 Update." (2002) *Arthritis Rheum.* 46, 2, 328–46.

40. Zhang, W. *et al.* (2008) "OARSI Recommendations for the Management of Hip and Knee Osteoarthritis, Part II: OARSI Evidence-Based, Expert Consensus Guidelines." *Osteoarthritis Cartilage.* 16, 2, 137–62.

41. Ottawa Panel. (2004) "Evidence-Based Clinical Practice Guidelines for Therapeutic Exercises in the Management of Rheumatoid Arthritis in Adults." *Phys Ther.* 84, 10, 934–72.

42. Youkhana, S. *et al.* (2016) "Yoga-Based Exercise Improves Balance and Mobility in People Aged 60 and Over: A Systematic Review and Meta-Analysis." *Age and Ageing.* 45, 1, 21–9.

43. Moonaz, S.H. *et al.* (2015) "Yoga in Sedentary Adults with Arthritis: Affects of a Randomized Controlled Pragmatic Trial." *J Rheumatol.* 42, 7, 1194–202.

44. Ornish, D. *et al.* (1990) "Can Lifestyle Changes Reverse Coronary Heart Disease? The Lifestyle Heart Trial." *The Lancet.* 336, 8708, 129–33.

45. Cohen D.L. *et al.* (2009) "Iyengar Yoga versus Enhanced Usual Care on Blood Pressure in Patients with Prehypertension to Stage I Hypertension: A Randomized Controlled Trial." *Evid Based Complement Alternat Med.*

46. Bernstein, A.M. *et al.* (2014) "Yoga in the Management of Overweight and Obesity." *American Journal of Lifestyle Medicine.* 8, 1, 33–41.

47. Halder, K. *et al.* (2015) "Age-Related Differences of Selected Hatha Yoga Practices on Anthropometric Characteristics, Muscular Strength and Flexibility of Healthy Individuals." *Int J Yoga.* 8, 1, 37–46.

48. Goncalves, L.C. *et al.* (2011) "Flexibility, Functional Autonomy and Quality of Life (QoL) in Elderly Yoga Practitioners." *Archives of Gerontology and Geriatrics.* 53, 2, 158–62.

49. *Ibid.* 42.

50. Hassett, A. L. and Clauw, D.J. (2010) "The Role of Stress in Rheumatic Diseases." *Arthritis Research and Therapy.* 12, 123, 1–2.

51. Wilson, D.B. *et al.* (2009) "The Association between Body Mass Index and Arthritis among US Adults: CDC's Surveillance Case Definition." *Preventing Chronic Disease.* 6, 2, A56.

52. Gabay, O. and Clouse, K.A. (2016) "Epigenetics of Cartilage Diseases." *Joint Bone Spine.* 83, 5, 491–4.

53. Dishman, R.K. (1982) "Compliance/Adherence in Health-Related Exercise." *Health Psychology.* 1, 237–67.

54. Bulent, O. *et al.* (2004) "Alterations in the Dynamics of Circulating Ghrelin, Adiponectin, and Leptin in Human Obesity." *PNAS.* 101, 28, 10434–9.

55. Barbour, K.E. *et al.* (2017) "Vital Signs: Prevalence of Doctor-Diagnosed Arthritis and Arthritis-Attributable Activity Limitation—United States, 2013–2015." *MMWR.* 66, 9, 246–5.

56. Barbour, K.E. *et al.* (2014) "Falls and Fall Injuries among Adults with Arthritis—United States, 2012." *CDC Weekly.* 63, 17, 379–83.

57. Centers for Disease Control and Prevention. (2016) "At a Glance Fact Sheets: Arthritis." Accessed May 23, 2018 at www.cdc.gov/chronicdisease/resources/publications/aag/arthritis.htm

58. Baker, C. (2018) "Briefing Paper: Obesity Statistics." *House of Commons Library.* 3336.

59. Centers for Disease Control and Prevention. (2011) "Arthritis as a Potential Barrier to Physical Activity Among Adults with Obesity—United States, 2007 and 2009." *MMWR.* 60, 19, 614–18.

60. Messier S.P. *et al.* (2005) "Weight Loss Reduces Knee-Joint Loads in Overweight and Obese Older Adults with Knee Osteoarthritis." *Arthritis Rheum.* 52, 7, 2026–32.

61. Bartlett, S.J. *et al.* (2004) "Small Weight Losses Can Yield Significant Improvements in Knee OA Symptoms." *Arthritis and Rheumatism.* 50, 9(S), S658.

62. Moonaz, S.H. *et al.* (2015) "Yoga in Sedentary Adults with Arthritis: Effects of a Randomized Controlled Pragmatic Trial." *J Rheumatol.* 42, 7, 1194–202.

63. Rioux, J.G. and Rittenbaugh, C. (2013) "Narrative Review of Yoga Intervention Clinical Trials Including Weight-Related Outcomes." *ltern Ther Health Med.* 19, 3, 32–46.

64. Arvonen, M. *et al.* (2016) "Gut Microbiota-Host Interactions and Juvenile Idiopathic Arthritis." *Pediatr Rheumatol Online J.* 14, 1, 44.

65. Scher, J.U. *et al.* (2015) "Decreased Bacterial Diversity Characterizes the Altered Gut Microbiota in Patients with Psoriatic Arthritis, Resembling Dysbiosis in Inflammatory Bowel Disease." *Arthritis Rheumatol.* 67, 1, 128–39.

66. Bravo, J.A. *et al.* (2011) "Ingestion of *Lactobacillus* Strain Regulates Emotional Behavior and Central GABA Receptor Expression in a Mouse via the Vagus Nerve." *Proc Natl Acad Sci USA.* 108, 16050–5.

67. Vanuytsel, T. *et al.* (2014) "Psychological Stress and Corticotropinreleasing Hormone Increase Intestinal Permeability in Humans by a Mast Cell-Dependent Mechanism." *Gut.* 63, 1293–9.

68. Cramer, H. *et al.* (2015) "The Safety of Yoga: A Systematic Review and Meta-Analysis of Randomized Controlled Trials." *Am J Epidemiol.* 182, 4, 281–93.

Chapter 5

69. Birch, S. (2012) "Sham Acupuncture Is Not a Placebo Treatment—Implications and Problems in Research." *Japanese Acupuncture and Moxibustion.* 8, 1, 4–8.

70. Hempel, S. *et al.* (2014) "Evidence Map of Acupuncture." Washington, DC: US Department of Veterans Affairs. Accessed June 18, 2018 at www.hsrd.research.va.gov/publications/esp

71. Oliver, M. (1992) "The Summer Day." From *New and Selected Poems.* Boston, MA: Beacon Press.

Chapter 6

72. Vgontzas, A.N., Bixler, E.O., and Chrousos, G.P. (2006) "Obesity-Related Sleepiness and Fatigue: The Role of the Stress System and Cytokines." *Ann N Y Acad Sci.* 1083, 329–44.

73. Ciriaco, M. *et al.* (2013) "Corticosteroid-Related Central Nervous System Side Effects." *J Pharmacol Pharmacother.* 4, 1, S94–S98.

74. Parmelee, P.A., Tighe, C.A., and Dautovich, N.D. (2015) "Sleep Disturbance in Osteoarthritis: Linkages with Pain, Disability, and Depressive Symptoms." *Arthritis Care Res (Hoboken).* 67, 3, 358–65.

75. Pollard, L.C. *et al.* (2006) "Fatigue in Rheumatoid Arthritis Reflects Pain, not Disease Activity." *Rheumatology (Oxford).* 45, 885–9.

76. Fishbain, D.A. *et al.* (2009) **"Does Pain Cause the Perception of Fatigue in Patients with Chronic Pain? Findings from Studies for Management of Diabetic Peripheral Neuropathic Pain with Duloxetine."** *Pain Pract.* 9, 5, 354–62.

77. Inoue, S. and Sluka, K. (2016) "Testosterone Protect against Development of Chronic Widespread Fatigue-Induced Muscle Pain." *Journal of Pain.* 17, 4, S68.

78. Chrousos, G.P. (2010) "The Hypothalamic-Pituitary-Adrenal Axis and Immune-Mediated Inflammation." *N Engl J Med.* 332, 1351–62.

79. Slavich G.M. and Irwin, M.R. (2014) "From Stress to Inflammation and Major Depressive Disorder: A Social Signal Transduction Theory of Depression." *Psychol Bull.* 140, 774–815.

80. Accessed at singlegalsguidetora.typepad.com on November 2, 2017.

81. Hewlett, S. *et al.* (2012) "'I'm Hurting, I Want to Kill Myself': Rheumatoid Arthritis Flare is More than a High Joint Count—An International Patient Perspective on Flare Where Medical Help Is Sought." Oxford: *Rheumatology.* 5, 1, 1, 69–76.

82. Louati, K. and Berenbaum, F. (2015) "Fatigue in Chronic Inflammation—A Link to Pain Pathways." *Arthritis Research and Therapy.* 17, 254.

83. Masson, C. (2011) "Rheumatoid Anemia." *Joint Bone Spine.* 78, 131–7.

84. Banks, W.A. and Erickson, M.A. (2010) "The Blood-Brain Barrier and Immune Function and Dysfunction." *Neurobiol Dis.* 37, 1, 26–32.

85. Dantzer, R. *et al.* (2014) "The Neuroimmune Basis of Fatigue." *Trends in Neurosciences.* 37, 1, 39–46.

86. Moonaz, S.H. *et al.* (2015) "Yoga in Sedentary Adults with Arthritis: Effects of a Randomized Controlled Pragmatic Trial." *J Rheumatol.* 42, 7, 1194–202.

87. Haaz, S. *et al.* (2008) "The Effect of Yoga on Clinical Parameters in Patients with Rheumatoid Arthritis." *Arthritis and Rheumatism.* 58, 9, S893.

88. Badsha, H. (2009) "The Benefits of Yoga for Rheumatoid Arthritis: Results of a Preliminary, Structured Eight-Week Program." *Rheumatol Int.* 29, 12, 1417–21.

89. Haaz, S. and Bartlett, S.J. (2011) "Yoga for Arthritis: A Scoping Review." *Rheum Dis Clin North Am.* 37, 1, 33–46.

90. Singh, V.K., Bhandari, R.B. and Rana, B.B. (2011) "Effect of Yogic Package on Rheumatoid Arthritis." *Indian J Physiol Pharmacol.* 55, 4, 329–35.

91. Evans, S. *et al.* (2013) "Impact of Iyengar Yoga on Quality of Life in Young Women with Rheumatoid Arthritis." *Clin J Pain.* 29, 11, 988–97.

92. Middleton, K.R. *et al.* (2017) "A Qualitative Approach Exploring the Acceptability of Yoga for Minorities Living with Arthritis: 'Where are the people who look like me?'" *Complementary Therapies in Medicine.* 31, 82–9.

Chapter 7

93. Hannan, M.T., Felson, D.T. and Pincus, T. (2000) "Analysis of the Discordance between Radiographic Changes and Knee Pain in Osteoarthritis of the knee." *Journal of Rheumatology*. 27, 6, 1513–17.

94. Bushnell, M.C., Ceko, M., and Low, L.A. (2013) "Cognitive and emotional control of pain and its disruption in chronic pain." *Nat Rev Neurosci*. 14, 7, 502–11.

95. Lamm, C., Decety, J., and Singer, T. (2011) "Meta-Analytic Evidence for Common and Distinct Neural Networks Associated with Directly Experienced Pain and Empathy for Pain." *Neuroimage*. 54, 2492–2502.

96. deCharms, R.C. *et al.* (2005) "Control over Brain Activation and Pain Learned by Using Real-Time Functional MRI." *Proc Natl Acad Sci USA*. 102, 18626–31.

97. Wager, T.D., Scott, D.J., and Zubieta, J.K. (2007) "Placebo Effects on Human μ-Opioid Activity during Pain." *Proc Natl Acad Sci USA*. 104, 11056–61.

98. Gwilym, S.E *et al.* (2009) "Psychophysical and Functional Imaging Evidence Supporting the Presence of Central Sensitization in a Cohort of Osteoarthritis Patients." *Arthritis Rheum*. 61: 1226–1234.

99. Lazar, S. *et al.* (2005) "Meditation Experience is Associated with Increased Cortical Thickness." *Neuroreport*, 16, 17, 1893.

100. Evers, A.W.M. *et al.* (2014) "Does Stress Affect the Joints? Daily Stressors, Stress Vulnerability, Immune and HPA Axis Activity, and Short-Term Disease and Symptom Fluctuations in Rheumatoid Arthritis." *Annals of the Rheumatic Diseases*. 73, 1683–8; Erfani, T. *et al.* (2015) "Psychological Factors and Pain Exacerbation in Knee Osteoarthritis: A Web-Based Case-Crossover Study." Sunnyvale: *Rheumatology*. S6, 005.

101. Zautra, A.J. and Smith, B.W. (2001) "Depression and Reactivity to Stress in Older Women with Rheumatoid Arthritis and Osteoarthritis." *Psychosom Med*. 63, 4, 687–96; Greco, C.M. *et al.* (2004) "Effects of a Stress-Reduction Program on Psychological Function, Pain, and Physical Function of Systemic Lupus Erythematosus Patients: A Randomized Controlled Trial." *Arthritis Care and Research*. 51, 4, 625–34; Goldenberg, D.L. *et al.* (1994) "A Controlled Study of a Stress-Reduction, Cognitive-Behavioral Treatment Program in Fibromyalgia." *Journal of Musculoskeletal Pain*. 2, 2, 3–66.

102. Russell, I.J. (2002) "The Promise of Substance P Inhibitors in Fibromyalgia." *Rheumatic Disease Clinics*. 28, 2, 329–42.

103. Sihvonen, R. *et al.* (2013) "Arthroscopic Partial Meniscectomy versus Sham Surgery for a Degenerative Meniscal Tear." *N Engl J Med*. 26, 369, 26, 2515–24.

104. Sihvonen, R. *et al.* (2018) "Arthroscopic Partial Meniscectomy versus Placebo Surgery for a Degenerative Meniscus Tear: A 2-Year Follow-Up of the Randomised Controlled Trial." *Ann Rheum Dis*. 77(2), 188–95.

105. Kaptchuk, T.J. (2002) "The Placebo Effect in Alternative Medicine: Can the Performance of a Healing Ritual Have Clinical Significance?" *Ann Intern Med*. 136, 11, 817–25; Snow, J. (2016) "Context Effects in Western Herbal Medicine: Fundamental to Effectiveness?" New York: *Explore*. 12, 1, 55–62; Walach, H. and Jonas, W.B. (2004) "Placebo Research: The Evidence Base for Harnessing Self-Healing Capacities. *Journal of Alternative and Complementary Medicine*. 10, Suppl 1, S103–12.

106. Bushnell, C.M., Ceko, M., and Low, L.A. (2013) "Cognitive and Emotional Control of Pain and Its Disruption in Chronic Pain." *Nat Rev Neurosci*. 14, 7, 502–11.

Chapter 8

107. Weinberger, M., Hiner, S.L., and Tierney, W.M. (1987) "Assessing Social Support in Elderly Adults." *Soc Sci Med*. 25, 9, 1049–55.

108. Zautra, A.J. and Smith, B.W. (2001) "Depression and Reactivity to Stress in Older Women with Rheumatoid Arthritis and Osteoarthritis." *Psychosom Med.* 63, 4, 687–96.

109. Keefe, F.J. and Caldwell, D.S. (1997) "Cognitive Behavioral Control of Arthritis Pain." *Med Clin North Am.* 81, 1, 277–90.

110. Center for Disease Control. (2017) "Depression Fact Sheet." Accessed October 26, 2017 at www.who.int/mediacentre/factsheets/fs369/en

111. Tak, S.H. and Laffrey, S.C. (2003) "Life Satisfaction and Its Correlates in Older Women with Osteoarthritis." *Orthop Nurs.* 22, 3, 182–9.

112. Gore, M. *et al.* (2011) "Clinical Comorbidities, Treatment Patterns and Direct Medical Costs of Patients with Osteoarthritis in Usual Care: A Retrospective Claims Database Analysis." *J Med Econ.* 14, 4, 497–507

113. Moonaz, S.H. et al. (2015) "Yoga in Sedentary Adults with Arthritis: Affects of a Randomized Controlled Pragmatic Trial." *J Rheumatol.* 42, 7, 1194–202; Middleton, K.R. *et al.* (2017) "A Qualitative Approach Exploring the Acceptability of Yoga for Minorities Living with Arthritis: 'Where are the people who look like me?'" *Complementary Therapies in Medicine.* 31, 82–9; Middleton, K.R. *et al.* (2018) "Feasibility and Assessment of Outcome Measures for Yoga as Self-Care for Minorities with Arthritis: A Pilot Study." *Pilot Feasibility Stud.* 4, 53.

114. Moonaz, S.H. *et al.* (2015) "Yoga in Sedentary Adults with Arthritis: Affects of a Randomized Controlled Pragmatic Trial." *J Rheumatol.* 42, 7, 1194–202.

115. *Ibid.* 114; Middleton, K.R. *et al.* (2017) "A Qualitative Approach Exploring the Acceptability of Yoga for Minorities Living with Arthritis: 'Where are the people who look like me?'" *Complementary Therapies in Medicine.* 31, 82–9; Middleton, K.R. *et al.* (2018) "Feasibility and Assessment of Outcome Measures for Yoga as Self-Care for Minorities with Arthritis: A Pilot Study." *Pilot Feasibility Stud.* 4, 53.

Chapter 9

116. Moonaz, S.H. *et al.* (2015) "Yoga in Sedentary Adults with Arthritis: Affects of a Randomized Controlled Pragmatic Trial." *J Rheumatol.* 42, 7, 1194–202; Middleton, K.R. *et al.* (2018) "Feasibility and Assessment of Outcome Measures for Yoga as Self-Care for Minorities with Arthritis: A Pilot Study." *Pilot Feasibility Stud.* 4, 53.

117. Satchidananda, S.S. (1990) *The Yoga Sutras of Patanjali.* Yogaville, VA: Integral Yoga Publications.

118. Listen to the full interview with Tina at www.youtube.com/watch?v=Z8S6_F7D2jo, accessed on November 2, 2017.

Chapter 10

119. McCauley, J. *et al.* (2008) "Daily Spiritual Experiences of Older Adults With and Without Arthritis and the Relationship to Health Outcomes." *Arthritis Rheum.* 59, 1, 122–8.

120. Norton, M.I. and Gino, F. (2014) "Rituals Alleviate Grieving for Loved Ones, Lovers, and Lotteries." *J Exp Psychol Gen.* 143, 1, 266–72.

121. Hobson, N.M., Devin, B., and Inzlicht, M. (2017) "Rituals Decrease the Neural Response to Performance Failure." *Peer J.* 5, e3363.

122. Li, S. *et al.* (2016) "Association of Religious Service Attendance with Mortality Among Women." *JAMA Intern Med.* 176, 6, 777–85.

123. Gore, M. *et al.* (2011) "Clinical Comorbidities, Treatment Patterns and Direct Medical Costs of Patients with Osteoarthritis in Usual Care: A Retrospective Claims Database Analysis." *J Med Econ*, 14, 4, 497–507.

124. Chang, K. *et al.* (2014) "Smoking and Rheumatoid Arthritis." *Int J Mol Sci.* 12, 22279–95.

125. *Ibid.* 120.

126. Bartlett, S.J. *et al.* (2003) "Spirituality, Wellbeing, and Quality of Life in Persons with Rheumatoid Arthritis." *Arthritis Rheum.* 49, 778–83.

127. Miller, W.R. and Rollnick, S. (2012) *Motivational Interviewing.* New York: Guilford Publications.

128. Mooventhan, A. and Khode, V. (2014) "Effect of Bhramari Pranayama and OM Chanting on Pulmonary Function in Healthy Individuals: A Prospective Randomized Control Trial." *Int J Yoga.* 7, 2, 104–10

129. Lazar, S. *et al.* (2005) "Meditation Experience is Associated with Increased Cortical Thickness." *Neuroreport*, 16, 17, 1893.

Chapter 11

130. You can see video instruction of this at www.youtube.com/watch?v=oVtnVwdIvkYn, accessed on November 2, 2017.

Chapter 13

131. Accessed at https://arthritis.yoga on November 2, 2017.